Case Management in Mental Health Services

Charlotte J. Sanborn is Assistant Professor of Clinical Psychiatry at Dartmouth Medical School, Director of Continuing Education at West Central Mental Health Services in Hanover, New Hampshire, and Director/Counselor of the Faculty/Staff Assistance Program at Dartmouth College. She has been active in the mental health movement for twenty years and has co-edited two books and authored or co-authored more than 35 articles on mental health. In addition to directing community mental health services in Hanover, Ms. Sanborn has served as a consultant to the National Institute of Mental Health, held office in various state and national medical records associations, and directed a Bi-State two-way closed circuit medical television network. She is currently President of the Association of New Hampshire Community Mental Health Agencies and Consulting Editor to the *Journal of Suicide and Life Threatening Behavior*. She is a board member of the American Association of Suicidology and lectures extensively on adolescent suicide.

Case Management in Mental Health Services

Edited by
Charlotte J. Sanborn

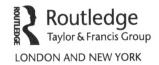

Routledge
Taylor & Francis Group

LONDON AND NEW YORK

Preparation of the following chapters was supported by government funding: "Case Management: A Remedy for Problems of Community Care" by Stephen S. Leavitt, "Case Management: Implications and Issues" by Michael L. Benjamin and Tal Ben-Dashan, and "The Experience in New York State" by Michael Ross, Nancy Riffer, and Tim Switalski. These chapters do not represent official policy of government agencies and/or institutions but rather those of the individual authors.

First published 1983 by The Haworth Press, Inc.

Published 2013 by Routledge
2 Park Square, Milton Park, Abingdon, Oxfordshire OX14 4RN
711 Third Avenue, New York, NY 10017

First issued in paperback 2015

Routledge is an imprint of the Taylor and Francis Group, an informa business

Library of Congress Cataloging in Publication Data
Main entry under title:

Case management in mental health services.

Bibliography: p.
1. Mentally ill—Care and treatment. 2. Chronically ill—Care and treatment. 3. Community mental health services. I. Sanborn, Charlotte J. [DNLM: Mental health services—Organization and administration. WM 30 C337]
RC480.53.C37 1982   362.2'0425   82-15495

ISBN 13: 978-1-138-87310-0 (pbk)
ISBN 13: 978-0-8665-6109-9 (hbk)

CONTENTS

Part VII

SUMMARY

FOREWORD

This is an important book. It addresses the crucial problem of the care and rehabilitation of the chronic mental patient. There are few who have worked in mental health who have not been impressed with the fact that despite our best efforts, intentions, and the most modern techniques there is a group of patients that require long-term care. They can no longer function as autonomous and self-sufficient individuals. The toll that these patients take in terms of effort and concern on the part of the family, professionals, and community resources is great. These are not exciting patients; they are difficult and draining of energy. Whether these patients are the products of institutionalization or, in large part, the cause of institutions, the patients with chronic mental illness have been present for centuries. Initially these patients wandered from village to village. Soon alm houses and poor houses became repositories for these individuals. In this country in the 19th century a great cry went up about the plight of the chronically mentally ill. Dorothea Dix and other reformers urged the states to empty the alm houses and develop state hospitals for the mentally ill with a county care plan for the chronic patient. In the early 1960s we saw the rise of the community mental health center movement as a reaction to these same state hospitals and with it the concept of the deinstitutionalization. This current movement has now brought us full circle with the return of the chronic patient to the community again, often going from village to village.

This book represents the most current attempt to facilitate the community care of the chronic patient. The chronic patient is seen, and often correctly so, without social and survival skills, surrounded and confronted by a maze of potentially helpful agencies and people. Frequently the chronic patient is left to negotiate these complexities alone, going from agency to agency, receiving fragmented care and assistance. In the face of these tasks the chronic patient often becomes increasingly frustrated, confused, and isolated with the only solution being the return to the institution. To prevent this circular process, the concept of the case manager has been developed. The case manager is supposed to provide a sustaining force for these patients.

The case manager provides continuity, assists in coordination of agency contacts, and aids the patient in problem solving. Through this sustained contact and the case manager's comprehensive knowledge of the individual patient, it is believed that the complexities of life facing the chronic patient can be simplified, and the goal for the chronic patient can be at best a productive life and at worst maintenance outside of an institution. Towards this effort this book serves as a valuable explication of the purpose of case management: the training, organizational and ethical issues of case management, and, even more valuable, reports of some actual experiences with varied ongoing case manager systems. The book serves as a useful document that discusses and delineates the basis for this new movement in community mental health. Most movements in community mental health have been pursued with an almost religious zeal motivated either by intense conviction or budgetary needs with their utility being determined only after the fact. This discussion of the case manager represents an opportunity to examine in detail many aspects of a new technique prior to total utilization. For this alone we are grateful to the contributors for the clear presentation of this new concept. In this sense the book is of seminal interest but should also provide a fertile ground for the planning of prospective studies of this new concept.

Gary J. Tucker, M.D.
Professor/Chairman
Department of Psychiatry
Dartmouth Medical School
Hanover, New Hampshire

CONTRIBUTORS

RICHARD F. ANTONAK, Ed.D.
Professor of Education
Coordinator, Developmental Disabilities Program
University of New Hampshire
Durham, New Hampshire

MICHAEL L. BENJAMIN, M.P.H.
Manpower and Development Specialist
National Institute of Mental Health
Washington, DC

MARK EISENSTADT, M.D.
Psychiatrist
Mystic Valley Mental Health Association, Inc.
186 Bedford Street
Lexington, Massachusetts

BRIAN FLYNN, Ed.D.
Mental Health Program Specialist
Department of Health, Education and Welfare
Region I, Public Health Service
Boston, Massachusetts

STEPHEN S. LEAVITT, M.D., Ph.D.
Medical Program Development Project
U.S. Department of Labor
Office of Workman's Compensation
Washington, DC

LINDA LYMAN
Thresholds, Incorporated
Chicago, Illinois

GARY MILLER, M.D.
Director, New Hampshire Division of Mental Health
Department of Health and Welfare
Concord, New Hampshire

SHARON MILLER, M.S.W.
Director, Office of Services Unification
Department of Mental Health
Lansing, Michigan

DAWN NELSON, M.Ed.
Mental Health Center of Southern New Hampshire
Derry, New Hampshire

HENRY E. PAYSON, M.D.
Professor of Psychiatry
Dartmouth Medical School
Hanover, New Hampshire

SANDRA PELLETIER, M.Ed.
Client Manager
Kimi Nicholas Development Center
Westville, New Hampshire

MICHAEL ROSS, Ph.D.
Program Director, Title XX Training
Office of Manpower/Development Training
Department of Mental Health
Albany, New York

THOMAS SALATIELLO, M.S.W.
Supervisor, Adult Services
New Hampshire Division of Welfare
Laconia, New Hampshire

TIM SWITALSKI
Office of Manpower/Development Training
Department of Mental Health
Albany, New York

GARY J. TUCKER, M.D.
Professor and Chairman
Department of Psychiatry
Dartmouth Medical School
Hanover, New Hampshire

DAVID WOLOWITZ, J.D.
Seacoast Office of New Hampshire
Legal Assistance
Lecturer on Law and Social Work
University of New Hampshire
Durham, New Hampshire

ACKNOWLEDGMENTS

I wish to gratefully acknowledge the contribution of each person who participated in this conference, especially Paul DellaRocco, the conference co-chairperson.

My special thanks to the moderators:

> Gary J. Tucker, M.D., Professor and Chairman, Department of Psychiatry, Dartmouth Medical School
>
> Jack Melton, Ph.D., Superintendent, Laconia State School and Training Center
>
> Bern Anderson, M.A., Director, Manpower and Training, New Hampshire Division of Mental Health and Developmental Services

This conference by the Department of Psychiatry at Dartmouth Medical School, the New Hampshire Division of Mental Health and Developmental Services and the Region #1 Office of the Department of Health, Education and Welfare was made possible in part through gifts from McNeil Laboratories and Pfizer Laboratories.

Finally, the complex task of running a conference and promoting attendance would not have been possible without an outstanding faculty combined with help from Judy Murphy, my secretary.

CJS

INTRODUCTION

From the inception of the community mental health center movement, the essence of the program has always been and will continue to be "to remove the locus of the care and treatment of the mentally ill from large custodial institutions to acute treatment in community-based facilities" that are responsible for and responsive to the needs of the people who live in those communities.

With the advent of that nine-syllable word "deinstitutionalization" and the "least restrictive alternative" phrase in the human services armamentarium, we all wondered what the newly bandied about term of "case manager" meant in relation to the professionals and the citizens themselves.

Because of these terms, the conference in the fall of 1979 at Waterville Valley was held to look at some of the issues that were of concern to a broad mix of people. These areas fell into the following categories as we saw them:

— Why Case Management?
— Organizational Issues
— Legal/Ethical Issues
— Training

We selected a faculty of local, regional, and national reputation to address these four topics in depth. This book is sectioned into parts that present "food for thought," examples of case management programs in the country within organizational structures, rehabilitation program models, different training models and approaches, questions of authority, funding, ethics, and legal rights as well as an historical overview of antecedents contributing to the present need for case management services.

Case management: What is "it?" Do we want/need "it?" Is this what to call "it?" Would we know "it" if we saw "it?"

The more we fully understand the context of case management as a human service reality, the greater will be our capacity to deliver a continuum of appropriate care to those in need.

We should take the contributions in this volume seriously. The idea that we ourselves may one (some) day find need for such services rarely crosses our minds. However, we are fallible, and we all have the responsibility to use our human skills—an important resource—so that each client and the population as a whole have an optimum chance for achieving a status of independent living.

Charlotte J. Sanborn

Case Management in Mental Health Services

Part I

WHY CASE MANAGEMENT?

Chapter 1

CASE MANAGEMENT:
THE ESSENTIAL SERVICE

Gary Miller, M.D.

We have heard a great deal about case management during the past four or five years. And it is no accident that our renewed interest in this essentially old-fashioned approach to service has coincided with the emergence of issues of critical nationwide significance in the mental health field. Few are now unaware of the plight of thousands of mentally handicapped people struggling to survive outside of institutions in our communities, and of the fact that our present service delivery system has not been effective in meeting the basic and special needs of many of these people.

During the late 1960s and the early 1970s, mental health workers placed great emphasis on moving people from the institutional to the community setting in the belief that patients would somehow benefit merely by virtue of their being "in the community." Reduction of institutional census was a major goal for state mental health systems and individual state hospitals. While the newly established community mental health centers made some inroads into the problems of chronic mental patients, little thought was given in those days by state agencies or the community programs as to whether and how communities could meet the overwhelming needs of these people who had spent many years of their lives in an institution which had demanded little of them and had fostered childlike dependency and atrophy of basic living skills. We now know that many of these individuals did not fare very well.

In January 1977, the General Accounting Office report on deinstitutionalization[1] called the attention of Congress to the tragedy of mentally disabled persons who had slipped through the cracks between the myriad of HEW agencies and their state and local counterparts. The President's Commission on Mental Health reported to the President in 1978 on the scope of the problem:

Time and again we have learned—from testimony, from inquiries, and from the reports of special task panels—of people with chronic mental disabilities who have been released from hospitals but who do not have the basic necessities of life. They lack adequate food, clothing or shelter. We have heard of woefully inadequate follow-up mental health and general medical care. And we have seen evidence that half the people released from large mental hospitals are being readmitted within a year of discharge. While not every individual can be treated within the community, many of the readmissions to the state hospitals could have been avoided if comprehensive assistance had existed within their communities.[2]

The census of institutions for the mentally retarded did not begin to fall as early, nor did it fall as rapidly, as that of state mental hospitals, but the trend is clearly in the direction of community care for most mentally retarded people.[3] Aside from some differences in nomenclature, e.g., substitution of the term normalization for deinstitutionalization, and of habilitation for rehabilitation, the needs and problems of the mentally retarded in the community are entirely comparable to those of the chronically mentally ill. As in the case of the chronically mentally ill, there are many mentally retarded people whose needs are not being met.[3]

The task panel on organization and structure of the President's Commission on Mental Health emphasized that the problems of deinstitutionalization are directly attributable to a lack of coordination and continuity in the delivery system:

> Panel members unanimously agreed that mental health services, even after 14 years following passage of the Community Mental Health Centers Act, were still fragmented, poorly coordinated, provided a narrow range of services which were often inappropriate to communities served, were plagued by the absence of continuity between state and local problems, and lacked a systematic approach to service delivery.[4]

In a similar vein, the General Accounting Office reported that "a coordinated system of care for the mentally ill through the CMHC program remains a goal rather than reality."[1]

In the light of these recent observations of the CMHC program, we should be aware that fragmentation and lack of coordination are not recently discovered problems, nor were they unanticipated in the early days of the community mental health movement. An analysis of then existing community mental health models published in 1964 by the Joint Information Service of the American Psychiatric Association and the National Association for Mental Health at the outset of the federal CMHC program specifically addressed the problem:

> The mentally ill . . . need a complete range of service if they are to have the best chance for recovery. But even in communities with highly developed services, individual agencies have tended to operate in isolation. As a consequence, there have been many serious gaps in service. Furthermore, it has been necessary for an individual to undergo a complete and separate interview and evaluation at each agency whose service he sought—a procedure wasteful of already inadequate professional time and disruptive and discouraging to the patient. It has also resulted in a given patient's being treated by a succession of different people.[5]

It was expected in 1964 that the new CMHC program would "coordinate existing programs . . . establish the missing elements in a single comprehensive service and . . . provide whatever . . . treatment is needed at the time it is needed and within the community where the patient lives."[5]

While the community mental health centers have greatly increased the variety and volume of service in hundreds of communities of the United States, the promise of 1964 has not been fulfilled, especially for those with chronic disability; weakened or absent family ties; excessive dependency needs; and a limited repertoire of personal, social, and vocational skills. It seems that the roster of essential services called for by the NIMH model of the community mental health center has lacked one key essential service.

Today, case management is recognized as one of the most essential services, if not *the* essential service, in community programs. It is viewed as a means of overcoming the complexity and fragmentation of our service system and of reaching the inadequately served chronically and severely disabled population.[6-11] Turner and TenHoor emphasize that "there must be *a single person (or team)* at the client level *responsible* for remaining in touch with the client on a continuing basis regardless of how many agencies get involved."[8] According to the Task Panel on Deinstitutionalization, Rehabilitation and Long-Term Care of the President's Commission on Mental Health, "Strategies focused solely on organizations are not enough. A human link is required. A case manager can provide this link and assist in assuring continuity of care and a coordinated program of services.''[12] The President's Commission on Mental Health accepted the recommendations of the Task Panel concerning case management and in turn recommended to the President that "state mental health authorities develop a case management system for each geographic service area within the state."[2] That should be accomplished, according to the Commission, through designation by the state mental health authority of one agency in each area to assume responsibility for case managing the chronically mentally ill of that area.[2] A similar mandate with respect to mentally retarded and other developmentally disabled persons issues from the current federal developmental disabilities legislation which establishes case management as a priority service.[13]

This degree of emphasis on case management is justified by evidence that it can work well. Its dramatic effectiveness in some settings suggests even that it may have been the missing element in the delivery system, the one "essential service" without which other resources and staff cannot successfully meet the needs of the more severely handicapped person.

Six years of research conducted by Leonard Stein, Mary Ann Test, and their colleagues in Madison, Wisconsin have established the effectiveness of case management in meeting the survival requirements of severely disabled and highly symptomatic people in a community setting.[7,14,15] Stein and Test have also shown that case management services must be maintained on an indefinite basis, for if the case managers are withdrawn from even relatively well-adjusted mental patients, their relapse and rehospitalization rates will rise, eventually approaching those of non-case managed controls.[14]

A federally funded project in Virginia, the Services Integration for Deinstitutionalization (SID) Project, demonstrated in both an urban and rural setting that case managers (called broker-advocates) can be effective in meeting the needs of chronic mental patients in the community.[16]

Weinman and Kleiner's case managers (called enablers) were successful in improving the social performance, self-esteem, and community tenure of former state hospital patients.[10]

Fountain House in New York City, which can be viewed as a case management program operated by former state hospital patients, has also been demonstrated to be effective in maintaining chronically disabled persons for long periods of time in the community.[17]

Whatever else we do to serve the severely disabled, chronically mentally ill, or mentally retarded person in the community, the evidence suggests that case management is a necessary ingredient. In the view of Norman Lourie, case management "is a vital, perhaps the most primary, device in management for any individual with disability where the requirements demand differential access to and use of various resources.''[11]

While it is tempting to regard case management as a new and revolutionary approach in mental health and mental retardation services, today's case management is in fact a model with numerous antecedents and analogues. It is a part of the history of the profession of social work. The vocational rehabilitation counselor who counsels and brokers services for his clients, the public health nurse and home health aide[18] who serve the client on his home turf all engage in activities related to case management. During the 1960s indigenous mental health workers employed by some community mental health programs performed in a fashion that would now be labeled case management.[19] One of the closest contemporary analogues of case management is the model of the family physician. His relationship to his patients and to his specialist colleagues closely resembles the relationship of the case manager to his clients and to categorical service programs.

We should not forget that the family is the prototype of case management. It is likely that far more sick and disabled people are case managed by their families than by all formal case management systems.[20] Fountain House in New York City and similar psychosocial rehabilitation programs such as Thresholds in Chicago and Horizon House in Philadelphia closely resemble the family in the support they provide to the disabled person.[21] A variant of case management may also be discerned in the activities of mutual help groups modeled on Alcoholics Anonymous.[22]

Given the tradition of case management in the human services and its current acceptability, it is not surprising that there are few mental health, mental retardation, or social services agencies today that do not subscribe to or claim to practice some form of case management. That fact should cause us to wonder what we are doing wrong. If everyone is doing case management, why do services to the severely handicapped remain uncoordinated and woefully inadequate? The crisis in our communities reported by the General Accounting Office and the President's Commission on Mental Health developed over a number of years during which case management activities were being carried out by service agencies throughout the country.

This dilemma suggests that significant problems remain in the way case management is defined and operationalized. As we have noted, case management activities are not new; they are as old as the helping professions and are currently being carried out in many programs. But these activities do not necessarily add up to a case management *system* such as that proposed by the National Institute of Mental Health,[8] the President's Commission on Mental Health,[2] and the American Psychiatric Association[23] as a remedy for the problems of the mentally handicapped in our communities.

It is important, therefore, that we distinguish between case management as a system and certain case management or case management-like activities which have come to be referred to simply as case management. The latter includes not only partial or fragmentary case management programs, but also some fairly traditional programs, such as intake and referral services, aftercare clinic programs and primary therapist assignments in outpatient clinics. For the remainder of this chapter, I will list and briefly describe a set of principles drawn in part from various recent approaches to and models of case management.[4,6,11,12,16,24-26] The principles are offered in an attempt to characterize the more global and systematic form of case management programs and activities which resemble, but are not, case management.

Principle 1. Case management should be conceptualized and implemented as a system. While the specific elements of case management are drawn from experience with a variety of models and approaches, case management is now being viewed as a major system. A case management system encompasses more than a set of activities or functions carried out by certain personnel on a part-time or full-time basis. Such functions as advocacy, brokerage, linkage, and referral have been carried out for many years by a variety of agencies and individuals and do not constitute, in and of themselves, a case management system. A case management system is not an ancillary or add-on service, nor is it a new therapeutic modality to be incorporated, without other modifications, into an existing mental health, mental retardation, or social service agency. It is a central theme of service delivery which required reconceptualization and probably reorganization of the entire delivery system of the agency. The following principles address the structure and content of the case management system.

Principle 2. A case management system must offer total case management regardless of the presence of partial case management programs or activities within or outside of the system. By total case management, I mean that the case manager is responsible and accountable for the well-being of the client at all times and regardless of whether the client is enrolled in specific service programs or housed in a facility. Total case management means simply that there is no buck-passing. The client cannot be transferred by the case manager to another agency or program. The case manager is responsible for meeting the client's needs, consistent with the mission of case management (Principle 6), through his own efforts or those of others. Involvement of others in the process, however, does not relieve the case manager of total responsibility. The term "referral," therefore, must be used with care in a case management system. The case manager does not relinquish responsibility, nor does he cease to be accountable, for the client when, through the referral process, another provider becomes involved. In a total case management system, it is appropriate that residents of state mental health and mental retardation facilities be assigned to community-based case managers before the individuals are returned to the community.[2]

Total case management is essential, because the disjointed case management activities carried out by a multiplicity of agencies at the local level (partial case management) increase the problems of fragmentation rather than resolve them.[11] These partial case management activities are so widespread that it is unrealistic to expect that every client will have only one case manager. What the system must assure, however, is that each client will have one case manager who assumes overall responsibility.

Principle 3. The total case management responsibility for a defined population, such as the chronically mentally ill, must be vested in a single agency at the local level. As the case manager is responsible for serving his clients, the system too must assume the responsibility for providing or securing the provision of all necessary services for the client population. One agency, therefore, must have the authority and responsibility for the case management system to insure proper management and coordination of the system in its service area and to reduce the inefficient use of resources.[27]

In a total case management system, it is important that personnel of the single responsible agency understand and appreciate the fact that the scope of responsibility of the agency's case managers is broader than that of service programs the agency may operate. If a community mental health center, for example, is the agency responsible for total case management of the chronically mentally ill, the case manager should be viewed as responsible for meeting the service needs of clients who have in common the fact that they have a mental disability. The case manager should not be viewed narrowly as a mental health case manager or as a provider of mental health services. Meeting the needs of chronically disabled people in the community will require that the case manager assemble an array of support services which extends substantially beyond the core clinical services traditionally provided by community mental health centers.[14,28,29]

Principle 4. The case management system is a management device for insuring accountability. The problems of the non-institutionalized mentally disabled population addressed by the President's Commission on Mental Health and the General Accounting Office are, at their root, management problems. The President's Commission called for "a much clearer delineation of responsibility and accountability for the care delivered to (the chronically mental ill) population."[2] According to the Comptroller General, one of the major causes of problems associated with deinstitutionalization is "the absence of an effective management system for clearly defining objectives, roles, responsibilities, actions to be taken, and monitoring and evaluation to be done by various agencies for effectively handling individual transitions from institutions to communities."[1]

Case management is the vehicle which can assure that services remain accountable to the client. Lucy Ozarin[30] opines that the "key words in case management are responsibility, continuity, and accountability." Accountability is obtained in a case management system by application of the concept of total case management (Principle 2) and by structuring the agency so that a significant number of its employees (case managers) are made responsible for clients rather than for performing certain functions or working in certain service locations. As the preliminary report of the President's Commission on Mental Health has stated, "the focus must be on people, not places."[31]

Some case management systems assign clients to teams of case managers rather than individuals, raising the issue of whether accountability can be maintained in such a system. Leonard Stein and Mary Ann Test feel that accountability is maintained and that staff burnout problems are reduced with a team case management model.[14] On the other hand, Lucy Ozarin contends that "responsibility and accountability are easier to fix when a single person is designated as a case manager."[30] There is less polarization on this issue than appears to be the case if we take into account the fact that even in the Stein and Test team model, one of the team members is the primary case manager for each patient. I think it reasonable to conclude, first, that from the viewpoint of the client, it is easier to relate to and hold accountable a single individual; second, that this does not preclude use of a team with total case management responsibility; and, finally, that any case management system must provide for rotating weekend and evening coverage, vacations, and other forms of temporary relief for individual case managers.

Principle 5. A case management system should be outcome oriented. The Task Panel on Organization and Structure of the President's Commission on Mental Health[4] observed that "at present services tend to become an end in themselves instead of a means to the end of improving the life functioning of consumers.'' The Task Panel recommended that ''service delivery mandates . . . be directed to objectives and outcomes rather than to specific service functions.'' This principle is especially important in case management systems, for it is not uncommon for case management to be reduced to a laundry list of roles, functions, and activities. The case management system must be oriented toward the achievement of specific goals for clients consistent with the mission of case management.

Principle 6. The mission of case management, and of the case management system, is to achieve the highest possible degree of personal growth, autonomy, and social performance of the client. Pursuit of this mission means that the case management system should provide as little as necessary to maintain the client's growth and social integration, avoiding doing for the client that which he is capable of doing for himself. It is important to recognize, therefore, that total case management responsibility does not require that the case manager smother the client with unwanted and unnecessary services. Achievement of maximum autonomy or self-reliance of the client calls for a delicate balancing act on the part of the case manager.[14,28,32] He must be available when needed, but at the same time, the case manager must gradually wean the client from total dependence on him and the support system.

As indicated by Principle 5 (outcome orientation), the activities of the case manager—brokerage, advocacy, counseling, linkage, referral, etc.— follow from the mission of case management and are not to be considered independent goals. I would like to say a word about one of these activities, advocacy, since the advocacy function in case management has generated some confusion and misunderstanding.

Leslie Scallett[33] is right when she says that ''advocacy is a word that comes loaded with conflict and connotations.'' It would be a serious mistake to regard the case manager's advocacy function as an element of an internal or external advocacy system for protecting the human and legal rights of the mentally disabled.[34] Formal advocacy systems based both within and outside of the state mental health agency are necessary, for the mentally disabled are subject to abuse, both intended and unintended, by institutions, neighbors, landlords, house parents, employers, and providers—including the case manager.

The case manager is certainly concerned with safeguarding the rights of his clients and will advocate on their behalf to secure those rights and obtain necessary services. As Wolfensberger has noted, however, the case manager's advocacy functions ''are really clinical service functions'' and ''as such, they are not free from conflict of interest.''[35] It is unfair to both the case manager and the client to expect the case manager to perform the functions of an advocacy system. In sum, the case manager is a service provider who, in pursuit of his mission, will be required to advocate on behalf of his client; but he is not, nor should he be considered, a legal advocate, ombudsman, or patient representative.[14]

Principle 7. The case manager must receive adequate training, backup, and support from the system. The tasks and responsibilities of a case manager in a total case management system are exceptionally demanding. The Task Panel on Deinstitutionalization, Rehabilitation, and Long-Term Care of the President's Commission on Mental Health outlined the scope of responsibilities of, and demands made upon, the case manager.

> (The case manager) should possess a variety of interpersonal skills, be familiar with the common difficulties of the chronically mentally disabled, and be knowledgeable about the community's resource system. The functions to be performed by a case manager include developing an individualized case management plan; monitoring and adapting it to the changing needs and circumstances of the chronically mentally disabled individual; and remaining in extended contact with the patient and acting as a friend and advocate as required and desired by him or her. The case manager must thus serve as the link between the chronically mentally disabled person and the complicated and fragmented service system and must be responsible for ensuring that the patient receives appropriate and high quality services in a timely fashion.[12]

Clearly, case management is not an office job; nor is it a nine to five job. And it certainly is not an easy job. The job description of a case manager covers a broader range of activities and responsibilities than that of most of today's professionals in the human services.

To meet these responsibilities, the case manager must have extensive initial training and continuing education in a variety of areas. He must also have the complete support and backup of his agency.

The agency must be structured so that the case manager has a sufficient degree of authority and status within the agency to carry out his mission. He is not merely a traffic cop who directs clients to the appropriate service. Case managers in Ozarin's words[30] are "responsible front line service providers." They must not be shackled by policies which restrict their latitude in making decisions on behalf of their clients. As in the family physician model, election of specialty services for clients is the responsibility of the case manager, not of the specialist.

The case manager's responsibilities also require that he has access to specialized consultation and technical assistance in areas related to the disabilities and problems of his clients. The agency should be structured to provide this capability.

Needless to say, agencies should strive to pay case managers a salary commensurate with their broad range of responsibilities.

Finally, the case load of a case manager must be held within reasonable limits to preserve the integrity of the system. Assignment by the agency of an extremely large number of disabled clients will jeopardize the case manager's ability to fulfill the mission of case management and may result in his burnout.

The point I have tried to make in this chapter is that a case management system is more than the hiring of case managers or the placing of a new box on the table of organization called "case management." If we are to cope effectively with the widespread problems of service program fragmentation and the unmet needs of developmentally disabled and chronic mental patients in the community, a case management system is required. In a case management system, a single case manager or case management team operating out of a single local agency assumes the total responsibility for and remains accountable for the personal well-being and social integration of those people who are clients of the system.

REFERENCES

1. *Returning the Mentally Disabled to the Community: Government Needs to Do More*, General Accounting Office, Washington, D.C., January 1977.

2. *Report to the President from the President's Commission on Mental Health*, Vol. 1, Washington, D.C., 1978.

3. M. Rosen, G. R. Clark, and M. S. Kivitz, *Habilitation of the Handicapped*, Baltimore, University Park Press, 1977.

4. "Report of the Task Panel on Organization and Structure," *Task Panel Reports Submitted to the President's Commission on Mental Health*, Vol. II, 1978, pp. 275–311.

5. R. M. Glasscote, D. S. Sanders, H. M. Forstenzer, and A. R. Foley, "A New Type of Health Facility. . . ," *The Community Mental Health Center: An Analysis of Existing Models*, The Joint Information Service of the American Psychiatric Association and the National Association for Mental Health, The American Psychiatric Association, 1964, pp. 1–11.

6. R. J. Gerhard, R. E. Dorgan, and D. G. Miles, *The Balanced Service System: A Mental Health Model of Social Integration*, 1979 (in press).

7. M. A. Test and L. I. Stein, "Training in Community Living: A Follow-Up Look at a Gold Award Program," *Hospital and Community Psychiatry*, Vol. 27, 1976, pp. 193–194.

8. J. C. Turner and W. J. TenHoor, "The NIMH Community Support Program: Pilot Approach to a Needed Social Reform," *Schizophrenia Bulletin*, NIMH, Vol. 4, 1978, pp. 319–344.

9. G. Golden, "Rehabilitation and Psychology," W. Neff (editor), *Rehabilitation Psychology,* American Psychological Association, 1971, pp. 168–200.

10. B. Weinman and R. J. Kleiner, "The Impact of Community Living and Community Member Intervention on the Adjustment of the Chronic Psychotic Patient," in L. I. Stein and M. A. Test (editors), *Alternatives to Mental Hospital Treatment,* New York, Plenum Press, 1978, pp. 139–159.

11. N. V. Lourie, "Case Management," *The Chronic Mental Patient: Problems, Solutions, and Recommendations for Public Policy,* American Psychiatric Association, Washington, D.C., 1978, pp. 159–164.

12. "Report of the Task Panel on Deinstitutionalization, Rehabilitation, and Long-Term Care," *Task Panel Reports Submitted to the President's Commission on Mental Health,* Vol. II, Washington, D.C., 1978, pp. 356–378.

13. Public Law 95-602, November 6, 1978, 95th Congress, "Rehabilitation, Comprehensive Services, and Developmental Disabilities Amendments of 1978."

14. L. I. Stein and M. A. Test, "An Alternative to Mental Hospital Treatment," in L. I. Stein and M. A. Test (editors), *Alternatives to Mental Hospital Treatment,* New York, Plenum Press, 1978, pp. 43–55.

15. M. A. Test and L. I. Stein, "Training in Community Living: Research Design and Results," in L. I. Stein and M. A. Test (editors), *Alternatives to Mental Hospital Treatment,* New York, Plenum Press, 1978, pp. 57–74.

16. *Service Integration for Deinstitutionalization, Final Report,* Rehabilitation Services Administration, Office of Human Development, H.E.W., Grant no. 15-P-55896/3, 1978.

17. M. A. Glasscote, "What Programs Work and What Programs Do Not Work for Chronic Mental Patients," in J. A. Talbott (editor), *The Chronic Mental Patient: Problems, Solutions, and Recommendations for a Public Policy,* American Psychiatric Association, Washington, D.C., 1978, pp. 75–85.

18. V. M. Sieder and C. J. Califf, *Homemaker-Home Health Aide Services to the Mentally Ill and Emotionally Disturbed: A Monograph,* National Council for Homemaker-Home Health Aide Services, Inc., New York, 1976.

19. E. F. Torrey, "The Case for the Indigenous Therapist," *Archives of General Psychiatry,* Vol. 20, 1969, pp. 365–372.

20. N. W. Bell and E. F. Vogel, Editors, *A Modern Introduction to the Family,* New York, The Free Press, 1968.

21. I. P. Robinault and M. Weisinger, "Selected Approaches to Psychosocial Rehabilitation," in I. P. Robinault and M. Weisinger (editors), *Mobilization of Community Resources, A Multi-Facet Model for Rehabilitation of Post-Hospitalized Mentally Ill,* ICD Rehabilitation and Research Center, New York, 1977, pp. 44–61.

22. P. R. Silverman, *Mutual Help Groups: A Guide for Mental Health Workers,* NIMH, Rockville, Maryland, 1978.

23. "Proposal for Public Policy on the Chronic Mental Patient," American Psychiatric Association Position Statement, in J. A. Talbott (editor), *The Chronic Mental Patient: Problems, Solutions and Recommendations for a Public Policy,* Washington, D.C., American Psychiatric Association, 1978, pp. 207–220.

24. M. A. Test and L. I. Stein, "Community Treatment of the Chronic Patient: Research Overview," *Schizophrenia Bulletin,* NIMH, Vol. 4, 1978, pp. 350–364.

25. *Principles for Accreditation of Community Mental Health Service Programs,* 2nd Ed., Joint Commission on Accreditation of Hospitals, Chicago, 1979.

26. J. E. Turner and S. Fine, et al., "Summary Report of Topic #1, Who Are the Chronic Mental Patients, Where Are They, and What Are Their Needs," Appendix D, in J. A. Talbott (editor), *The Chronic Mental Patient: Problems, Solutions, and Recommendations for a Public Policy,* Washington, D.C., American Psychiatric Association, 1978, pp. 231–237.

27. T. D. Glenn, "Exploring 'Responsibility' for Chronic Mental Patients in the Community," J. A. Talbott (editor), *The Chronic Mental Patient: Problems, Solutions, and Rec-*

ommendations for a Public Policy, Washington, D.C., American Psychiatric Association, 1978, pp. 173–193.

28. R. H. Lamb, "Guiding Principles for Community Survival," in R. H. Lamb (editor), *Community Survival for Long-Term Patients*, San Francisco, Jossey-Bass, 1976, pp. 1–13.

29. R. H. Lamb, "Acquiring Social Competence," in R. H. Lamb (editor), *Community Survival for Long-Term Patients*, San Francisco, Jossey-Bass, 1976, pp. 115–129.

30. L. D. Ozarin, "The Pros and Cons of Case Management," in J. A. Talbott (editor), *The Chronic Mental Patient: Problems, Solutions, and Recommendations for a Public Policy*, Washington, D.C., American Psychiatric Association, 1978, pp. 165–170.

31. "Preliminary Report of the President's Commission on Mental Health," quoted in Report of the Task Panel on Deinstitutionalization, Rehabilitation, and Long-Term Care, *Task Panel Reports Submitted to the President's Commission on Mental Health*, Vol. II, Washington, D.C., 1978, pp. 356–378.

32. G. W. Fairweather, D. H. Sanders, D. L. Cressler, et al., *Community Life for the Mentally Ill - An Alternative to Institutional Care*, Chicago, Aldine Publishing Company, 1969.

33. L. Scallett, "Advocacy is a Loaded Word," *Proceedings: Symposium on Safeguarding the Rights of Recipients of Mental Health Services*, NIMH, 1977, pp. 8–9.

34. J. P. Wilson, H. A. Beyer, and B. Yudowitz, "Advocacy for the Mentally Disabled," in L. E. Kopolow and Helene Bloom (editors), *Mental Health Advocacy: An Emerging Force in Consumers' Rights*, NIMH, 1977, pp. 3–15.

35. W. Wolfensberger, "A Model for a Balanced Multicomponent Advocacy/Protective Services Schema," in L. E. Kopolow and Helene Bloom (editors), *Mental Health Advocacy: An Emerging Force in Consumers' Rights*, NIMH, 1977, pp. 16–35.

Chapter 2

CASE MANAGEMENT:
A REMEDY FOR PROBLEMS
OF COMMUNITY CARE

Stephen S. Leavitt, M.D.

Introduction: The "Third Revolution"

The October 1977 issue of *Psychiatric Annals* was devoted to a debate about what Dr. Milton Greenblatt labeled the "third" revolution in mental health. The first was defined as the period of moral treatment of the 18th and 19th centuries; the second, as the Freudian enlightenment of the first half of the 20th century. The third revolution was defined as the community mental health revolution. The essence of this revolution lay in (1) concern for total community mental health and (2) organization and delivery of services on a community base.

Other articles in the issue debated the question of whether the third revolution should be defined as pharmacological or socio-political. The pharmacological argument stated that the revolution, which brought with it deinstitutionalization of the mentally ill, resulted primarily from the introduction of chlorpromazine and related drugs. The social argument asserted that the transition of the mentally ill from large hospitals to the community was due to the evolution of such transitional facilities as halfway houses, day treatment centers, cooperative apartments, home treatment programs, outpatient satellites, and after care services.

The truth, of course, lies somewhere in between. Aaron Lazare postulates that there are presently four conceptual models for the treatment and management of the mentally ill. The schizophrenic client gets medication, implying a biological etiology; undergoes psychotherapy, implying that past experience affects his present dysfunction; may be subject to token economies, indicating that behavior can be shaped by reinforcement; and is a member of a therapeutic community meant to reintegrate him into society.[1]

Community Care: Theoretical Basis and Practical Problems

The theoretical and practical basis for community treatment of the mentally ill arises from a growing understanding of the deleterious effects of institutionalization of human function and some perception of the growth potential of mentally ill clients treated in the appropriate community setting. While individuals with major mental disabilities are at risk for experiencing progressive deterioration of social function, this deterioration can be prevented to some degree by structured opportunities for meaningful, responsible activity.[2] Although individuals with severe mental disabilities are not easily able to apply social or economic skills learned in one setting to another, they are able to function, given sufficient social support.[3]

From a practical point of view, however, the integration of biological, psychotherapeutic, behavioral, social, and economic forces into a coherent system of service which is organized to match the needs of individual clients has been difficult to achieve on a large scale.

Problems of community care for the chronically mentally ill are as well known as the rationale for endorsing community care. The problems include service fragmentation, poor coordination, a narrow and inappropriate range of services, and lack of systematic approaches to service delivery.[4] Mental health agencies experience serious difficulties over the issues of legitimacy and boundaries.[5] Additionally, there is often no fixed point of responsibility for the achievement of client goals. Numerous agencies with their own financial, professional, political, and administrative pressures operate independently and thus prevent any successful integration of services.[6]

California's Invisible System of Community Care[7]

California provides a dramatic example of the difficulties inherent in the shift of the locus of responsibility for mental health services from a state hospital system to the community. In 1957 the entire system consisted primarily of ten state hospitals with outpatient continuing care provided by the State Bureau of Social Work. Now the program is run primarily by 58 counties. In 1957, 98% of the state budget was spent on state hospitals. Now only 30% is spent on state hospitals and 70% on county programs. Over that same period of time, the combination of effects—tranquilizing drugs, state funding of county programs, aid to the totally disabled, and increases in state reimbursement of county programs—has been associated with a decline in the population of state hospitals from 32,000 to a little more than 5,000 as of 1979.

During this same period, however, the mental health program as a "system" of operating elements, each related to the next through predetermined objectives, rules, inputs, and outputs, has become fragmented and, for the most part, invisible to those policy-makers who would like to determine the program's effectiveness and rationally allocate money for its support. A typical large county program has 30 discrete, often competing, cost centers and 15 or more physical locations. In contrast to the ready availability of information concerning the extent of institutionalization under the state hospital system, the community system has lost track of institutionalization because of the diversity and number of facilities in which the chronically mentally ill can be institutionalized outside of state hospitals. Finally, in contrast to the state hospital system, the community treatment system, because of the diversity of funding sources, does not easily lend itself to fiscal analysis. Presently, in California only 37% of the estimated $913 million in public mental health expenditure can be accounted for in the "mental health program budget."

The invisible mental health system has raised serious questions—not only for policy-makers who cannot establish clear objectives and set rational budgets, but also for its clients. The primary client issues are: (1) the rise of non-hospital institutionalization in nursing homes and in board and care facilities; (2) the capacity of the system to allocate appropriately services to specific target populations such as the elderly, children, and minorities; (3) the use and misuse of commitment laws to manage clients in the community; and (4) the quality and uniformity of treatment services.

Case Management: A Remedy for Problems of Community Care for the Chronically Mentally Ill

Case management is being offered as a remedy for many of the problems of community care. In the *Principles of Accreditation of Community Mental Health Service Programs*, case management is described in the following way:

> Case management services are activities aimed at linking the service system to a consumer and at coordinating the various system components in order to achieve a successful outcome. The objective of case management is continuity of services . . . Case management is essentially a problem solving function designed to ensure continuity of

service and to overcome systems rigidity, fragmented service, misutilization of certain facilities, and inaccessibility.[8]

This definition addresses most of the ills of community treatment systems. Problems of accessibility are addressed through the activity of linking services to consumers. Problems of poor continuity of care are covered in the "coordination activity." The nature of the professional activity involved is clearly defined as "problem solving."

The implementation of case management in a county, however, poses issues of definition and methodology which must be clarified if case management—as a problem-solving function—is to be applied in a real setting, and, if applied, to achieve any affect other than further fragmenting program operation or simply adding to the list of interested agencies to which the mentally ill client must be accountable. These issues involve the concept of management itself, the case management mission, the nature of case management decisions, and the role of case management agencies in the community. While case management has been described as a problem-solving function, it is not immediately obvious what constitutes a problem, how it gets solved, who should solve it, and precisely how community-wide "systems" problems—rigidity, fragmented service, etc.—can be overcome by the activities of a case manager.

In the design of a case management system for the Continuing Care Services Section of the County of California, many of these issues were explored. Some were solved; some still await solution.

Sacramento County's Continuum of Community Services

When the California legislature passed its historic commitment reform law in 1967-68 thereby accelerating the movement of patients from state hospitals to communities, Sacramento County had few local resources. Almost half of the patients who were admitted to the county hospital were transferred to the state hospital. The Sutter Hospital received an NIMH Community Mental Health Center grant, but otherwise there were no public outpatient services. The Sacramento County 5-year plan noted that there were no 24-hour emergency and crisis intervention services in the county, no public treatment programs for children and adolescents, and no neighborhood services.

The county responded vigorously to this situation and attempted to develop a network of community-based services to provide a continuum of services for those patients coming into the community from the state hospital and those patients entering directly into community care from emergency room or other sources. Thus by 1975 for this 700,000 person county, the number of hospital admissions had dropped from 1200 in 1969 to less than 100 in 1974. At the same time outpatient admissions rose from 10,000 to well over 100,000.[9]

A diversified set of community resources was established. In 1977 these included intensive care facilities, sub acute facilities, 24-hour crisis clinics, mental health treatment centers, transition living facilities, enriched residential facilities, board and care homes, locations for independent living, and services to provide transportation and referral.[10]

Case Management Design Project: Sacramento County

As the continuum of care grew, the problems of fragmentation, inadequate coordination, lack of continuity between the state and the local service system, and unsystematic service delivery began to attain more visibility. Some of the problems were that agencies "closed-in" on themselves and pursued their own interests and the interests of their selected client group at the expense of the mentally ill population as a whole. Planning, service delivery, assessment, communication, and resource sharing were poorly coordinated. There were discontinuities in service delivery (clients fell through the cracks). Decision making was unsystematic, and there was inadequate assurance that the level of care being provided was proper.

The county staff concluded that case management could help considerably in resolving these difficulties. The county had acquired a continuing care services section made up of social workers and social work assistants from the state. Once this group of case workers was in place, development of a case management system became a priority mission.

The case management development project involved the following five overall tasks performed over an 18-month period:

Task One: Survey of community facilities and cases
Task Two: Definition of objectives
Task Three: Establishment of a system for case management decisions
Task Four: Development of case management tools
Task Five: Development of a case management record system and a new organizational structure

The result of the effort is contained in the *Case Management Agency System Handbook Designed for Sacramento County.*[11]

Analysis and Data Gathering: Toward a Definition of Case Management

It was clear from the outset that while the staff recognized the need for a number of improvements in service delivery and coordination, they were unfamiliar with standard management concepts and practices; hence, they could not visualize how to translate their clinical insights into action which might effect community decisions. The initial work in the project therefore focused on individual and workshop activities to define problems and objectives and to bridge the gap between case management of an individual client and case management as a community function.

Case management was defined as the process by which managers could assure that resources were obtained and utilized effectively and efficiently in the accomplishment of the program's objectives. The objectives of the case management program which together constituted its mission were to be based on the clinical needs of individual clients as well as the needs of target populations.

The Case Management Mission

In reaching their definitions of case management, the staff immediately recognized the need to be more precise regarding their mission as it might apply to an individual case or to an entire case load. The final description of mission was based upon data from several sources. Workshops with the case management staff and with community agencies personnel were held to identify their perception of outcome for different types of clients. Similarly, interviews with clients in hospital, board and care, and office settings were conducted to identify client perceptions of successful and unsuccessful outcome. Finally, an analysis of the agencies' 500 case records was conducted. The survey determined the distribution of clients by problem characteristics and services provided to them.

In the survey of cases, it was noted that the acting-out and recidivist population had 40% more problems with medications than the population overall and 300% more behavior problems; yet they received significantly less service from case workers and agencies than did easier-to-handle clients. They got 50–60% less monitoring of medication and 20% less activity addressed at linking them with outside programs. Hence, one aspect of the mission was to allocate services to clients most in need of support rather than to those who were most tractable or attractive.

Second, information concerning the use of medication and the effectiveness of treatment programs was sparse. In addition the pattern of treatment data showed that more was known about the chronic tractable population than about the population showing either high potential for growth or high potential for rehospitalization and acting out. For all populations, it was desirable to monitor the effectiveness of treatment or social programs as well as the nature of such interventions. Hence, the case management mission included not only service, but evaluation.

Third, it was recognized that there were vast differences in the population served in terms of age, level of impairment, risk of disability, potential for anti-social behavior or potential for growth. In contrast to the diversity of the population served, the existing administrative and professional operations of the staff did not include parallel differences in the allocation of staff time, skills, experience, or function. Hence, another case management mission was to redefine the case management organization in such a way that there was a better match between patient problems and the utilization of staff resources than before.

Fourth, the case management mission did not assume that existing services were the best ones, nor that the case management team's only mission was to facilitate use of the present system. Because of its access to data from a wide population and because it was in contact with all services, organizations, and resources effecting clients, the case management staff felt it was appropriate for it to monitor constantly the emerging needs of its client population and evaluate them against the existing and proposed programs being developed in the community. The case management mission hence included planning for new resources and recommended modifications of existing service based on data drawn from its client population.

Fifth, the case management staff recognized that there were barriers to independent living. Agencies would rather hold onto "good" clients rather than risk getting "bad" ones. Clients themselves often appeared to deteriorate after they had made successful steps toward independence. Likewise, the economic and social supports of the community care system often did not reward leaving the system. Instead the system often compounded the psychological tasks of independent living with added economic and social stressors. Case management needed to facilitate the transition outward by anticipating the crises associated with growing autonomy.

Sixth, the staff recognized that the traditional effects of labeling clients and focusing attention on client problems rather than assets and on client defects rather than skills tended to perpetuate the self-fulfilling prophecy that, once labeled, mentally ill clients would remain in the system or return. One case management mission was to undercut this phenomenon by balancing the focus on impairment with the recognition of a client's potential for growth.

With these issues in mind, the staff agreed that the *mission of case management should be to assure for each client the best possible opportunity for independent community living*. This mission was the same as for that of the community care system as a whole. The mission provided a basis for systematic decision making and appropriate allocation of staff resources.

Case Management Decisions

Case management decisions were defined as those decisions, made by case managers, the outcome of which would determine whether or not the client had been provided the best possible opportunity for independent community living. The boundaries of case management decisions were identified as these:

1. If decisions were based on an overestimation of the client's capacity to function, it was quite possible that his or her potential for independent living would be limited when, as a result of a failure at attempting independence, the client was returned to an unnecessarily restrictive environment—one which corresponded with behavior born from crisis rather than behavior resulting from a gradual attempt to master environmental demands.

2. If decisions were based on an underestimation of the client's capacity to function, it was possible that his or her potential for independent living would be limited because environmental demands for developing or improving technical or social skills of living were too low to stimulate growth.

Recognizing the importance of case management decisions and the difficulty in reaching correct decisions, the case management system needed to contain checks and balances and to be iterative in structure. The checks and balances were obtained by establishing not one, but a series of evaluative perspectives for the case manager to utilize when assessing an individual client. The iterative structure referred to a desired step-by-step quality in case management monitoring—this quality was achieved through setting short-term goals and monitoring for results shortly before results were to occur.

Twelve basic questions, each leading to alternative decisions, were identified. These questions deal with the client, his/her present environment, needed environmental changes, and methods for effecting an appropriate linkage between the client and the community. They are listed separately in Table 1.

Table 1

Case Management Questions

1. How do I best match a client with an environment in the community? (An environment includes residential, treatment, socialization, and, for some clients, vocational support services.)

2. How can I identify an environmental unmet need; that is a needed environmental element which might improve this client's chance for independent living or at least improve the client's chance for reaching a "highest possible" level of function?

3. What factors should I evaluate to judge a client's risk or potential for disability? A client may have been disabled due to mental illness, but appears relatively functional today. More data than that from a recent interview may be necessary to understand whether I am dealing with a client who could be potentially severely impaired.

4. How frequently and with what intensity does this client need to be followed to prevent recidivism or to optimize the potential for growth?

5. On what basis might I set a date for status review? What factors might I wish to consider if my action is to prevent a cyclical or otherwise foreseen problem?

6. What kind of systems interventions (or services) should be provided to this client? A system intervention in behalf of a client is one which links the client to a resource, guides the transition from one resource to another, finds resources, and assesses needs or results.

7. What kinds of personal interventions are appropriate? A personal intervention is based on the personal relationship between client and case manager. Most social workers can provide brief reality testing; can meet with families and clarify communications, set behavioral goals; conduct psychotherapeutic groups; arrange for placement of clients in

Table 1 (*continued*)

programs; set appointments and follow up; and establish a long-term personal relationship with the client.

8. What combination of systems and personal intervention should be provided for this client, which will also result in allocation efforts in the best interests of *all* clients?

9. How do I set goals for a client? What is the baseline for setting a goal? What are goals?

10. What information should be recorded in the file?

11. What are my information needs for this client from agencies, residences, and treatment personnel to monitor properly progress and prevent recidivism?

12. What approach might be taken to introduce this client to new programs in the community? What, for example, do board and care home or program operators need to know in order to assist the client in reaching his/her growth potential?

Data for Case Management Decisions

Case management of individuals and populations depends upon a method for uniform, accurate, reliable, and balanced assessment of clients and their present or potential environment.

Uniformity denotes wide agreement on definitions and methods of observation. *Accuracy* requires that *observations* of client behavior be based upon an adequate set of variables and that these variables be properly graded. *Reliability* refers to the capacity of observers in the system to produce similar observations. Finally, a *balances assessment* was one which utilized client skills and assets equally with client symptoms and liabilities to establish service goals and plans.

The case manager's assessment resources include past information derived from hospital records, agency histories, court records, and the history as presented by the client. This information provides the case manager a basis for assessing the client's strengths and potential for getting into trouble. The interview with the client provides the best source of information regarding the client's present status, and in many cases it will give the case manager the best insight into the client's potential strengths. The client's perspective of his/her environment and the support systems presently in place can be utilized by the case manager to determine the need for changes in physical environment, social contact, or therapeutic support. Information from therapists, friends of the client, and other agency personnel will round out the picture and help the case manager to evaluate his/her own observations.

Risk, Stress and Stressors, Potential for Growth, and Steps Toward Autonomy

A systematic and iterative approach to case management decision depended—it was concluded—upon the case manager's capacity to address four critical issues about the client and his/her environment. These issues included those regarding risk, stress, potential for growth, and steps toward autonomy. These four concepts will be described below in brief. With each description, we have included key assessment characteristics which can assist the case manager in defining these issues:

Risk

Risk is the chance that an event such as an episode of mental illness will occur. Usually the event is of serious nature, such as death, accident, property loss, monetary loss, hospitalization, etc. Insurance companies refer to individuals covered by a policy as risks, indicating that the individual, or organization, or piece of property has a potential for some mishap or liability. In mental health the use of the term is almost exactly the same. A mentally ill client is at risk or has a potential for acting-out—unsafe behavior; for impairment—becoming psychotic; and/or for utilizing intensive and costly medical treatment facilities—such as acute hospitals. The nature of risk is described by the potential consequences. In the mental health treatment system, clients confront the risks of:

— grave disability
— property damage
— injury to other
— injury to self
— hospitalization

Prediction and evaluation.   Risk is predicted on the basis of history (or experience) and the existing factors which could modify the likelihood of the occurrence of the event, be it acting out or disability. Predictions become more accurate when there is greater knowledge of the client and his/her environment.

Risk for hospitalization, for example, goes up with the following assessment characteristics:

1. Acuteness of present mental illness episode.
2. Severity of mental illness episode.
3. Recidivism rate.
4. History of institutionalization.
5. Severity of acting out behavior.
6. Power of operating stressors (to be discussed later).

Risk is offset by the following assessment characteristics:

1. History of moderate to good levels of response to mental health treatment.
2. Social assets.
3. Potential for improvement in social, intellectual, or emotional skills.
4. Present social, intellectual, or emotional skills.

Risk can also be offset if:

1. The case manager has detailed knowledge of the client's past response to stressors; particularly if severe mental illness episodes were known to be triggered by specific stressors.
2. The case manager has knowledge of future stressors.
3. The client has the capacity to report changes in his/her condition.
4. There is evidence that the client in the past has been able to utilize effectively the mental health treatment system to modify the impact of stressor events.

Stress and Stressors

Stressors refer to external events in the life of a client which are known to precipitate emotional symptoms or which are likely to precipitate symptoms in the future. Knowledge of these is essential to prevention. Prevention includes education, anticipatory guidance, crisis intervention, changing the client environment, and other techniques, e.g., planned regression. Note that the word stressor is used rather than stress. Stress depicts an individual's response; a stressor is the observable cause of stress. The categories of stressors are indicated in Table 2.

Table 2

Stressors

a. Stressors or crises due to losses of persons: Severity is greater when the personal loss comes after a long and emotional important relationship. Emotional importance is *not* limited to positive relationships. Death of a spouse has been shown to be the most stressful crisis in western civilization. Death of a parent may be equally stressful.

b. Stressors or crises due to losses of physical function: Severity is greater as the resulting impairment increases. Physical functions are lost as a result of aging. Loss of ovarian function, loss of function due to stroke or heart failure are stresses associated with the aging process. Injury and illnesses also create life stress.

c. Stressors associated with residential change: These stresses are greater as they entail greater social disorganization and reorganization. Movement from a state hospital to the community constitutes a stress associated with complete reorganization of an individual's life plus personal losses.

d. Stressors associated with changes in the social support system: These include changes in finance, employment, and socialization groups.

e. Stressors associated with changes in the mental health treatment systems: These include change of physician, changes in medication, in socialization programs and other therapists.

f. Stressors associated with changes in legal status: These include changes with reference to participation in the mental health system, such as going from voluntary to involuntary treatment or leaving conservatorship. Others could be receiving traffic tickets or involvement with litigation.

g. Stressors related to social isolation or deprivation: These occur when individuals are found living in a withdrawn state without adequate stimulation.

h. Miscellaneous stressors such as good fortune, falling in love, marriage, pregnancy, job promotion, etc.

Assessment of stressors.   Based on interview and information from records and relevant others in the client's environment, the case manager should be able to compile an inventory of client stressors. For each of the stressors, the following should be considered:

1. What are the specific characteristics of the stressor, e.g., persons involved, circumstances, etc.?
2. To what degree *did* this stressor or *might* this stressor impact the client's capacity to function? Degrees can be indicated as: (1) Minimal—client's responses were or will be only subjective. There was or would be no significant change in function. (2) Moderate—client's responses are subjective. There was or would be change in function, but not sufficient to require any degree of social disorganization; or reorganization. (3) Severe—client responses warrant change in social structure or regimen, such as increased medication, counseling, increased frequency or appointment with therapist. There was or is apt to be change in social ties and some minimal acting out behavior. (4) Very severe—if unattended by caretaker or therapist, stressor did or would result in client regression and/or severe acting out behavior; client might well require hospitalization.
3. To what degree is client able to anticipate and report development of stressor event? (1) Not at all. (2) Possibly if asked. (3) Will indicate clearly that trouble is brewing. (4) Will independently seek help.
4. What prescription is recommended for managing stressor event in the future for this client?

Potential for Growth

Growth. Increase in an individual's coping capabilities. The increase can manifest itself anywhere on a continuum from mastery of a basic skill necessary for daily activity—e.g., proper hygiene—to the application of skill and judgment to reach a complex, important managerial decision.

The individual's potential for growth rises when his/her physical and social environment has the following characteristics[12]:

1. An environmental situation in which physiological needs are fulfilled—i.e., food, clothing, and shelter.
2. A residential environment in which there is safety from abuse and property damage.
3. A positive and effective mental health treatment program where the client demonstrates acceptance and appropriate utilization of treatment resources.
4. A social support system outside the mental health treatment setting in which the client's role and contribution is clear and in which needs for a clear role and/or a sense of belonging are fulfilled.

5. Evidence that the client's social support system has the capacity to enhance the client's self-esteem through recognition and reward.
6. An environment—including social support system—requiring the client to learn to solve problems, and to make decisions in the activities of daily living, time management, money management, and matters of aesthetics and personal taste.

The individual's potential for growth falls when:

1. There is no recent history (past five years) of successful growth or problem solving.
2. The individual has a high percentage of institutionalization—closed system living.
3. Manifestations of mental illness include depression and immobility.
4. There is no recent history (five years) indicating the capacity *to desire* to learn and accomplish new skills.
5. Social and problem-solving skills at interview are low.

The potential for growth will increase if:

1. The client demonstrates the capacity to ask for help and effectively communicate needs and emotions.
2. The client has features that can attract the interest and concern of others.
3. The client has a history of seeking and achieving intimacy in personal relationships.

Steps Toward Autonomy

Autonomy refers to the capability of *self-control* and *self-direction*. It refers to the capacity to make ethical decisions and live according to the dictates of one's own perceptions and reason.

The mentally ill client becomes autonomous through the acquisition and application of skills or capabilities. While the potential for growth must be present through the establishment of a suitable environment and social support system, achievement of capabilities for independent living also demands the learning or relearning of specific skills. These skills can be classified according to the following categories:

1. Self-care
2. Safety

3. Transportation
4. Illness management
5. Money management
6. Time management
7. Interpersonal skills
8. Aesthetic and athletic skills
9. Vocational skills

Table 3 illustrates those skills necessary to achieve independence in the community.

Table 3

Skill List

Skills or Self-care for:

- Hygiene (self)
- Nutrition (self)
- Toilet
- Dress and appearance
- Cooking
- Cleaning
- Decorating, maintenance of personal possessions
- Maintenance (cleanliness and hygiene) of personal space—room, apartment

Safety Skills

- Ability to recognize unsafe behavior—improper disposal of cigarettes and matches, smoking in bed
- Ability to prevent unsafe behavior in self or others
- Capacity to respond to unsafe conditions through appropriate reporting and simple action—use of fire extinguisher, telephone to police, etc.
- Capacity to recognize felonious behavior or plans and not participate—stealing, rape, arson, forgery
- Capacity to get help in case of attack or molestation

Skills of Illness Management

- Appropriate use and understanding of medication
- Recognition of developing symptoms and signs of illness

Table 3 (continued)

- Capacity for self-referral
- Capacity to participate in psychosocial therapies

Money Management Skills

- Recognize and count currency, make change
- Negotiate the purchase of items
- Account for purchases
- Maintain simple records of income
- Maintain simple records of expenses
- Make periodic payments on time and within budget
- Compare values—shop

Time Management Skills

- Follow routine without supervision
- Plan daily routines of increasing variety
- Carry out daily plan
- Plan weekly and monthly routines and execute them

Transportation Skills

- Capacity to determine orientation in progressively complex physical environment—building, neighborhood, town
- Map reading (optional)
- Capacity to lay a course between two points
- Capacity to follow directions for travel
- Capacity to give directions for transportation by another person
- Capacity to utilize public transportation
- Capacity to drive

Interpersonal Skills

- Capacity to introduce self
- Capacity to describe self
- Capacity to engage in general conversation
- Initiate and carry out simple to complex negotiations
- Organize small to large group activities
- Share responsibilities with other persons
- Accept reward and recognition from others
- Give recognition and appreciation to others
- Engage and disengage from a group activity

Table 3 (continued)

- Disengage from one person and initiate contact with another
- Share intimate thoughts and feeling (ideals, hopes, plans, fears, wishes)
- Initiate sexual behavior–disengage or modify sexual advances
- Engage in sexual intimacy

Aesthetic and Athletic Skills

- Recognize the nature and use of media—paint, clay, leather, plants, etc.
- Copy a design
- Create a design
- Follow the design
- Evaluate the strengths and weakness of artistic products
- Teach artistic activity
- Participate in athletic conditioning
- Learn rules of athletic games
- Participate in athletic games
- Teach athletic games

Vocational Skills

- Follow orders from production of a product or provisions of a service, on a continuum from close supervision to without supervision
- Learn job skill from on-the-job observation
- Learn job skill from reading and apply skill
- Prepare a resume of past work
- Participate in an employment interview
- Provide continuous employment services
- Supervise others in the work place
- Train others

Establishing a Match between Client Need and Environmental Resources: The Last Step in Case Management

Establishing a link between client needs and environment resources is the end product of the case manager's training, skill, and efforts at assessment. The first phase of this activity is analysis of information gathered during assessments. The second phase—which is dependent upon the resources available in the specific community with which the case manager is working—is the assignment of the client to one of a number of service categories.

Service Categories

Service categories were developed to describe the level of case management effort appropriate to various categories of client's needs. Low levels of effort were clearly appropriate for clients who were (1) stable and (2) already independent. High levels of case management are necessary for unstable clients at risk for severe behavior problems. Service categories, accordingly, go from "no service" to a "therapeutic assignment." See Table 4.

Factors in the Service Category Assignments

Seven general factors were identified for consideration in planning the service category assignment. These are stability, forthcoming stressors, potential disability, potential for growth, "maintenance" requirements, cyclical disturbances, and client independence. These factors are somewhat interrelated.

Stability vs. Instability. If the client's condition is unstable, the service assignment must be geared to follow progress toward stability. While issues of potential for growth and potential severity are relevant, the truly unstable client will require reassessment shortly after stabilization.

Forthcoming Stressors

Service assignments should correspond to the impact of forthcoming stressor events on a client. The level of case management activity should be intensified prior to a crisis point in a client's life.

Client Potential Disability

Even after an immediate crisis has been resolved, the client's potential for disability may remain high. Case management activity will clearly be related to this risk.

Client Potential for Growth

It may take some months to develop an optimum environment for client growth and establish a workable schedule for assessment and goal attainment. During the period prior to establishing a final plan, case manage-

Table 4

Service Categories

No Service	Assessment and Information Services Only	Assessment and Monitoring	Assessment, Monitoring and Program Linkage
Simplifications of no action are that the client can manage his/her own affairs and can recover from the inevitable errors in judgment that occur in everyone's life. It is essential to distinguish doing nothing from disregard or bureaucratic disinvolvement. The implication of no-action is that the client can ask for help or consultation—a highly adaptive response to stress. The implication of "denial of the application" or bureaucratic unavailability is quite the opposite in that it fosters helplessness in the client. Name and file kept for statistical purposes only. This group may contain individuals whose disability is not due to mental illness alone, but to social and economic difficulties. Often they will be directed to other agencies.	These clients include those who for one reason or another have received case management assessment. The category can include prepetition screenings and certifications where the client does not fall into another service category. Assessment services can include a complete case management evaluation. Individuals in this category can also be given cards to contact case managers if necessary and can be provided education on mental health resources in the community. The decision made by the case management team is the date—if any is appropriate—for another assessment. The critical question in reaching this decision is—What if no case management services are provided? What risk is involved? From these considerations will come a time frame for a next assessment.	Client plans are developed for monitoring changes with regard to employment, therapy, finance, and legal status. Clients in a wide variety of low risk-growth and "maintenance" categories fall into this service level. Such individuals have often received more services—at a higher service category—at one time, and the service category is lowered in light of greater independence. Management scenarios should revolve around crisis intervention and prevention. Evaluation of these cases should include client stressors. Case reviews should be planned to anticipate predicted stressors—such as return to work, movement to a new location, discharge from a conservatorship. Upon contact, the case manager should first establish the client's status overall with regard to employment activities, therapy, finance, etc. Inquiry should be made with regard to the forthcoming stressor event, such as its imminence, plans, support, and changes in client behavior, perceptions and emotional control which may indicate deterioration in function	Program linkage and monitoring requires the following steps: a. Assessment of the client and his/her resources. b. Identifying community resources and programs which provide the client a continuum of life support and opportunities for reinforcement and instruction in social, intellectual and emotional skills. c. Preparation of referral letters to relevant community resources. d. Assurance that the client actually becomes engaged in the community resource programs in question. e. Development of a monitoring plan through which the case management team can receive information on client behavior and progress from the community—such as deterioration in appearance, increase in manifestations of mental illness, failure to attend clinics and sessions. Psychiatrists and other therapists are the primary focus of day-to-day management for these clients. The case manager is responsible only for tracking progress, assuring the stability of program linkage, setting dates for new contacts, arranging for referral information, and establishing review and reassessment dates.

Table 4 (continued)

Direct Service Assignment	Therapeutic Team Assignment	Assessment and Monitoring (Cont.)	Assessment, Monitoring and Program Linkage (Cont.)
In addition to assessment, monitoring, and program linkage, certain clients will be assigned to direct case management therapeutic services. The basis for this assignment is: 1. there is clear need for the service. 2. the service is not available in the community and/or that 3. case management personnel have particular expertise and knowledge The direct services mentioned here include ongoing, face-to-face, therapeutic efforts with the client for development of skills. As opposed to monitoring and program linkage services, these direct services are akin to psychotherapy. They include scheduled counselling services, crisis intervention sessions (more than one or two), group therapy, family therapy, etc. The client may also have another therapist and participate in other programs.	For selected clients—high risk, adolescents—with client's therapeutic treatment team. The worker will furnish program linkage and monitoring services as well as other functions to facilitate communication among members of the treatment team. Case managers providing this category of service will probably be known to other treatment personnel in the community such as psychiatrists, conservator, family members, hospital staff members, and others. These managers will facilitate clear, unambiguous communication among the treatment team members in addition to providing program linkage and other services.	Careful step-by-step planning and increased therapeutic efforts may support the individual during the period of transition. Individuals in this service category are expected to manage their own program linkage. They can be provided education by the case management team, but appointments, phone calls, and letters of introduction to community resource programs are not required. **On-Call Service Assignment** Selected clients—high risk, unstable, cyclical—will require on-call services. These clients will be best assigned to special teams geared to manage on-call problems.	Included in this category are services including: 1. Placement in facilities 2. Establishment of contact with SSI **Service Refusal** Clients who refuse case management services are given a separate category. The role of the case manager is to determine the need for civil action to attain involuntary treatment services for such clients. Hence, the service refusal category of clients has two classes: 1. Clients who refuse services, but are *neither* gravely disabled, nor a danger to themselves or others. 2. Clients who refuse services and who fulfill criteria for involuntary mental health treatment.

ment activity may need to be more intense than after the optimum environment has been established.

So-Called "Maintenance" or "Sustenance" Cases

Individuals in this category are in an optimum environment for their growth potential when assessment of client *skills* and mental illness process indicates that, beyond the present level of autonomy, the client's capacity for developing new capabilities will be limited. The major function of case management activity for such clients will be preventive. Data will be required to anticipate stressors which may increase the client's potential for disability or to alert the treatment system to increases in the client's level of impairment. Periodic evaluation of medication may also be appropriate.

The Cyclical Client

Such clients may require different levels of case management intensity over time. Periods of on-call management may be required during periods of excitement or depression.

The Independent Client

The principle of no action or minimal case management action may be most appropriate to clients with low levels of impairment whose environment is adequate for the development of skills for independent living.

Case Management Beyond the "Group Practice of Social Work"

Concurrent with the development of a design for decision making for the individual case was the establishment of a mission and strategy through which the agency could impact the use and development of community resources. This effort was of critical importance in permitting case management actually to remedy the problems of community care. During the project, the staff defined the transition of a social work agency to case management as moving from the "group practice of social work" to operation of a case management system.

The strategy to implement the case management agency required the development of new capabilities. These included record keeping, community resource assessment, data and policy analysis, and planning. The case management agency strategy is illustrated in Table 5.

Table 5

Case Management Agency Strategy

- To know the number of citizens fitting the target population.
- To provide this population information about and access to case management services.
- To provide any member of this population an equitable assessment of his/her present and potential capacity for independent living.
- To provide an individualized and equitable program of case management and other services to these individuals based on their needs in reaching an optimal status of independent living.
- To know the number and nature of community resources available to this population which can assist in the activities of independent community living.
- To know the number and nature of community resources which are *known to be effective* in assisting such a population in the activities of independent living needed by this population based on the assessment of present clients but unavailable in the community. To provide such information on a periodic basis to those responsible for community mental health programs.
- To seek actively and develop needed community resources to meet unmet needs and to provide necessary education and guidance to existing community resources to improve their adequacy or efficiency.
- To evaluate the success of the agency's mission on the basis of statistically sound case review, feedback from community agencies and mental health consumers, and data from the literature.

Summary and Discussion

With the transfer of mental health treatment from state hospitals to communities have come greater opportunities for reintegration of mentally ill clients into the community and concomitant problems. These problems—fragmentation of service, lack of accountability for outcome, reinstitutionalization, and potentially increasing costs—require the development of a community facility whose function is assuring that adequate resources are provided to mentally ill clients in the community.

Case management has been identified as a method of improving the coordination and delivery of services in the community. The definition of case management proposed by the Joint Commission on Accreditation of Hospitals indicates that case management should exist to facilitate the use of existing community resources and pursue outcome objectives presumably existing in community mental health programs.

Experience in the design of a case management system for implementation in the county of a Sacramento, however, indicates that case management agencies, if they are to be truly effective and if they are not to become simply another agency to which the mentally ill client is accountable, must take a more assertive and self-directed role than proposed in the Commission's definition.

Case management must be defined as the process by which community resources are identified and allocated to achieve program objectives. The mission of case management is to assure for each client and for the target population as a whole that there is an *optimum chance* for achieving a status of independent living.

Such a mission identified by the Sacramento County staff provided the basis for identifying case management decisions. These decisions—about the client and the environment in which he/she lives—in turn depend upon the assessment of the client's capability to live independently.

Because the population of the mentally ill is diverse in demographic characteristics, in risk, in potential for growth, and in susceptibility to crisis, case management services must be based upon the analysis of client needs.

The case is made for a system of assessment which gives equal weight to client growth potential and client deficiencies. Parallel to these categories of client strength and weakness are categories of service ranging from "no service" to monitoring and tracking activities to continuous "on-call services."

The transition from the "group practice of social work" to case management agency requires a specific strategy, new skills, and new capabilities for its staff. With these in place, case management may well fulfill its role in supporting community care of the mentally ill.

If case management agencies do not take a planning initiative and do not develop tools to translate their knowledge of clients' needs into realities in the mental health system, they will not be able to strengthen the system of community care. Worse still, case management will become no more than a non-judicial conservator for the mentally ill.

REFERENCES

1. A. Stone, "Response to the Presidential Address," *The American Journal of Psychiatry*, Vol. 136, No. 8, 1979, p. 1020.

2. J. Strauss and W. Carpenter, "The Prediction of Outcome in Schizophrenia," *Archives of General Psychiatry*, Vo. 27, 1972, pp. 739–746.

3. R. Carkhuff and F. Berenson, *Teaching as Treatment*, Amherst, HRD Press, 1979.

4. D. Miles, *"Implementation of a Balanced System of Services, A Report on the Experiences of the Northeast Georgia Mental Health/Mental Retardation Consortium,"* Georgia Department of Human Resources, 1977.

5. L. Bachrach, *Deinstitutionalization: An Analytical Review and Sociological Perspective*, U.S. Department of HEW, Public Health Service NIMH, No. (ADM) 76-351, 1976, p. 24.

6. *Old Problems New Directions*, the 1978/1979 Budget Augmentation for Mental Health, presented by Edmund G. Brown, Governor, Health and Welfare Agency, Department of Health, Mental Health Program, State of California.

7. California Assembly Permanent Subcommittee on Mental Health and Developmental Disabilities, Leona H. Egeland, Chairwoman, *Improving California's Mental Health System: Policy Making and Management in the Invisible System*, Berkeley, California, Teknekron, Inc., 1979.

8. *Principles for Accreditation of Community Mental Health Service Programs*, Accreditation Council for Psychiatric Facilities, Joint Commission on Accreditation of Hospitals, 1976, pp. 20–21.

9. R. Yarvis and D. Langsley, "Do Community Mental Health Centers Under Serve Psychiatric Individuals?", *Hospital and Community Psychiatry*, Vol. 29, No. 6, 1978.

10. J. Barter, L. McMahan, and C. Foland, *Development of Community Based Services: Leaving the Institution Behind*, Sacramento County Mental Health Department, 1977.

11. *Case Management Agency System Handbook Designed for Sacramento County Department of Mental Health*, Berkeley, California, Teknekron, Inc., 1978.

12. c.f. Maslow, Abraham, "A Theory of Human Motivation," *Psychological Review*, Vol. 50, pp. 370–396. This and other work provide relevant theoretical considerations.

Chapter 3

CASE MANAGEMENT:
IMPLICATIONS AND ISSUES

Michael L. Benjamin, M.P.H.
Tal Ben-Dashan, M.A.

In recent years, as the deinstitutionalized chronically mentally disabled have attempted to reintegrate into less restrictive community settings, their needs as well as the obstacles they have encountered in the human service delivery system have been enumerated extensively in the scientific literature and by service providers in the field. Any discussion of case management, its desirability and necessity, must, therefore, be placed within a context which provides both an historical and current perspective on the needs of the chronically mentally disabled as well as the organizational developments, characteristics, and nature of the service delivery system.

Since the early 1960s, national policy as well as approaches toward the treatment of the mentally ill in the United States have changed considerably. The growing availability of effective psychoactive drugs, new forms of psychotherapy, and the mounting concern for public health and preventive measures, as well as the emphasis at the time on general social welfare, sparked an interest in community-based psychiatric care. Great attention was paid to social and institutional factors and their impact on health and individual functioning. This emerging spirit and commitment to community-based mental health programs was embodied in President Kennedy's address on Mental Illness and Mental Retardation of 1963 and the Community Mental Health Centers Act to which it gave rise. The Act presaged a major shift in the locus of care for the chronically mentally ill. Beginning in the mid-1950s, deinstitutionalization of patients, from distant and crowded state mental hospitals into community settings across the nation, dominated the mental health service ideology.

Approximately a decade following the burgeoning of the community mental health movement and deinstitutionalization, as the optimism of the 1960s and early 1970s gave way to a more conservative social climate, these efforts have been criticized and condemned. Community mental health centers are charged with having failed to accept and develop services to meet the needs of the chronically mentally ill. Communities are increasingly resentful of unplanned discharges and the housing of patients in their midst. Legal and judicial pressures on the system to safeguard patient rights have intensified and the nation's federal policy-makers agree that a coherent policy toward the severely mentally disabled is lacking.[2,12]

These developments, coupled with a growing public awareness of the substandard living conditions of the deinstitutionalized in the community, have pointed to the critical nature of the situation and have given rise to a reassessment of service delivery modes. As the President's Commission on Mental Health and the Community Support Program initiative undertaken by the National Institute of Mental Health indicate, the needs and experiences of the chronically mentally disabled are being documented, evaluated, and analyzed.[7,12]

The mentally disabled, specifically those individuals with severe or persistent mental or emotional disorders that seriously limit their functional capacities, possess a number of significant characteristics. These range from individual/personal factors, such as impaired capacity in performing basic activities of daily living and meeting basic life needs to interpersonal difficulties due to a frequent lack of motivation and/or ability to seek help from or sustain rapport with human service workers as well as extreme dependency on others. Lastly, treatment factors, such as sustained contact with the mental health system and the need for treatment other than acute short-term intervention, are characteristic of the chronically mentally disabled.[8,9] These functional attributes clearly point to outstanding areas of need. As Turner has stated "like the general population, mentally disabled adults need food, clothing, housing, medical care, transportation, education, recreation and money."[9] Aside from these very basic human needs, the chronically mentally disabled have some unique and critical needs These include assistance in applying for income, medical and other benefits, 24-hour crisis assistance, psychosocial rehabilitation, supportive services of indefinite duration, such as supportive work opportunities and living arrangements, as well as medical and mental health care.[9,11,12]

Given this broad spectrum of needs, a number of significant problems and issues inherent in the service delivery system and in local communities have come to the fore. These factors have emerged since meeting and providing for the needs of the chronically mentally disabled require the efforts of multiple agencies and service providers as well as community acceptance. The lack of appropriate services, coordination accountability and continuity in service delivery; fragmentation; and the questionable quality of care provided are some of the issues related to the service delivery system. Community resistance and opposition are related to issues of the chronically mentally disabled in the greater community. Financial and fiscal factors and legal issues have also been identified.[1,12]

The growing awareness of such fundamental deficiencies has given rise to the development of a number of conceptual frameworks which aim to address some of these obstacles and to increase commitment to programs that attempt to provide for the wide range of needs presented by this population and to rehabilitation and social support which are crucial to successful functioning of the chronically mentally disabled in the community. These approaches include the Balanced Service System, Natural Networks System, and the Community Support System, among others.

The federally funded Community Support Program specifically directs its efforts toward stimulating states across the nation to plan and provide for appropriate services for the severely mentally disabled adult. The Program outlined ten components of a Community Support System necessary for meeting the needs of this target population. Case management has been identified as one of these essential components. In the past year and a half, 19 states and the District of Columbia have contracted with the National Institute of Mental Health to develop community support systems. Case management approaches have been developed and implemented in many of these states and interest in this service mode continues to increase.[6].

A recent assessment of these initial experiences and a preliminary review of the literature, undertaken by the Center for State Mental Health Manpower Development at the National Institute of Mental Health, have indicated that case management poses complex conceptual and operational difficulties. It has also become clear that the effective implementation of case management has far-reaching implications not only for mental health services but for the service delivery system as a whole.[3]

As the literature and service providers in the field attempt to define and develop frameworks for case management, a wide range of case management roles and functions are being advanced. It has become apparent that many of these approaches are unsystematic and lacking in specificity. However, a number of general trends have emerged, and factors which affect the design and implementation of case management have been identified.

Case management on the *client level* is broadly perceived within the context of traditional casework; that is to say, case management functions outlined most often include assessment, planning, linking, monitoring, advocacy, and direct service delivery. Beyond this initial definitional stage, the specifications of roles and tasks within each of these broad functional categories vary significantly and range from the abstract to the particular. As a result, a fully developed framework for case management, with detailed role and function specifications, has yet to be presented. It is clear, therefore, that there is a growing need for programs and service planners to approach case management more systematically and analytically and to consider some, if not all, of the factors outlined in this paper.

1. Case management within the service delivery system. If case management is to be effective in meeting the needs of the chronically mentally disabled, it must be perceived as a component within the larger service system—a component which attempts to alleviate *some, not all,* of the imperfections which are inherent in that system. Thus, certain system-wide functions need to be performed if case management is to succeed. These functions ought to be viewed at least on two levels, the client or direct service level and the agency or administrative level. Case management on the client level should be defined rather narrowly and specifically and should consist of linking the necessary basic services, e.g., intake, assessment, planning, referral, and follow-up, so as to tie together the provision of services to the client. These functions should focus on the client and his/her needs and should have fairly immediate and direct results.

On the other hand, functions at the agency level ought to provide for administrative linkages which integrate service agencies and providers and enable the case manager to cross multiple agency boundaries. The process of developing such linkages would involve resource and program development, joint programming and planning, interagency agreements, and so on. In other words, case management will not be effective if the case manager is not only charged with meeting the client's direct service needs but also with "filling in the gaps" in the service delivery system. Resource and program development and community advocacy are extremely complex and time-consuming. If they are to be dealt with successfully, they must be accomplished by an individual or agency with the wherewithal, i.e., power, mandate, funding, to perform such tasks. That is not to say that the case manager should not be responsible for advocating on a face-to-face and client-to-client basis or for creatively utilizing existing resources to provide for the needs of the client. The case manager ought to be accountable for coordinating the service plan and for identifying service gaps but should not be expected to deal with these deficiencies on his/her own. In short, administrative and client-level functions must be realistic, clearly delineated, and separated and must be performed in tandem if case management is to benefit the client.

2. Organizational and structural issues. The development of a series of standardized, predictable, and accountable interagency agreements which will enable the case manager to act as the designated point of accountability for service provision is a key organizational issue. A necessary step in achieving this is the assessment of the nature of the service delivery system present at each setting in order to specify type and range of interagency agreements needed. These agreements serve a variety of purposes. They heighten the awareness of shared responsibilities as well as problems through formal public agreements and procedures. They provide, moreover, formal recognition of those individuals, i.e., case managers, engaged in "boundary-spanning" activities as the appropriate, legitimate personnel to perform these tasks. Interagency agreements serve to routinize the paths between organizations and through contractual arrangements, they provide redress and back-up procedures for case managers to resolve differences encountered.

A number of additional critical organizational and structural questions need to be asked if case management is to address appropriate systems issues:

a. To what extent do duplication, fragmentation, and overlap exist between service systems and of what negative consequence are they for clients?
b. What range of services will be used by case managers in the course of service provision?
c. What problems have been reported by workers attempting to secure resources in the past?
d. What is the level of complexity of negotiating tasks performed by those in case management positions?[5]
e. Are highly skilled workers performing simple tasks far below their level of expertise?
f. What staffing patterns are possible?
g. What case management model is optimal given available resources and organizational limitations?
   — Individual versus Team?
   — Psychosocial versus Medical?
h. What level of authority will be given to case managers seeking to obtain resources for clients?
i. What level of authority is needed?

j. What is the perception of those in administrative or supervisory positions as to the appropriate range and emphasis of tasks to be performed by case managers?

3. Manpower/personnel issues. Because of the limited information about the total range of tasks actually performed in the delivery of case management, precise statements with regard to what knowledge/skill/ ability mix is necessary to perform such tasks cannot be made. However, the following questions should prove useful:

a. What is the content of case management activities?
b. What skill areas prove particularly important? What knowledge areas? What abilities are used?
c. Does the job design of the case management model entail conflicting demands for service provision to clients, accountability to the agency, and mandates to provide linking, coordinative, and advocacy functions? Which role predominates?[5]
d. How can the manpower resource allocation patterns be utilized optimally?

4. Funding issues. A careful review of the current financing for care of chronic mentally ill adults leads to the conclusion that funding is a major problem area.[8] At the federal and state levels, efforts should be initiated to look at the possibilities of correcting those regulations and legislation that now prevent reimbursement specifically for case management function. Local service providers should communicate specifics about federal and state regulations which serve as disincentives for case management.

5. Evaluation issues. One of the weaknesses of the literature on case management is the lack of data on the performance of case management functions by the case manager. What is required is a systematic examination of various definitions of case management and of the conceptual framework on which they are based, with special emphasis on the provision of services to the chronically mentally ill. An indicator of success would be improved client access to services.

6. Training/manpower development issues. One of the barriers to curriculum design and development is the lack of an agreed upon definition of case management. The ideas related to case management grew out of day-to-day practice needs; consequently, the development of the conceptual framework lagged far behind. Until the development of a clearer definition of case management and a logical framework around existing ideas related to case management takes place, curriculum design, training package development, and assessment of existing manpower will occur on a less-than-adequate basis.

7. *Political/legislative considerations.* Legislative support can be a double-edged sword. Case management has received increased attention in recent years as specific mandates incorporated in various federal laws regarding human services have indicated. The P.L. 93-516 (Rehabilitation Act) requires that each consumer be served based on an Individualized Written Rehabilitation Plan. Similarly, an individualized plan of one kind or another is required or encouraged by other legislation such as P.L. 93-647 (Social Services - Title XX), P.L. 94-142 (Education for All the Handicapped Act), P.L. 94-223 (Medicaid - Title XIX), and P.L. 95-602 (Developmentally Disabled Assistance Act). These approaches all imply or specifically require case management. However, case management is rarely defined in operational terms. The proposed Mental Health Systems Act incorporates requirements for establishing further accountability in service delivery by mandating the development of a case management system in providing for chronically mentally ill. Unfortunately, the existence of these multiple mandates has resulted, in many respects, in continued confusion and ambiguity regarding case management—which agency(ies) actually should take the lead and be held accountable, how responsibilities may best be fixed, and how various agencies who provide case management should interact within the service delivery system.

It is evident that other political factors exist which may impinge on the implementation of case management in a particular agency/locality. These factors would vary from state to state, community to community, and agency to agency. Needless to say, the impact of these factors on the delivery of services should not be underestimated.

Conclusion

With the growing recognition of case management as a necessary service mode in the provision of services to various targeted populations and with the accumulation of experiential and scientific information, case management has been offered as a ''cure-all'' for the difficulties encountered by disabled clients as they attempt to integrate into community life. This chapter has argued that case management for the chronically mentally disabled is a complicated concept to define and implement and an approach which has far reaching implications for the service delivery system. Case management, therefore, must not be perceived as a panacea for addressing the imperfections of the service delivery system. Instead, case management should be viewed in a specific context as one of a number of essential components within a system which aims to assist the chronically mentally disabled in achieving adequate functioning in the community.

REFERENCES

1. L.L. Bachrach, "Deinstitutionalization: An Analytical Review and Sociological Perspective," NIMH Series D, #4, 1976.

2. T. Ben-Dashan, "Mental Health Care in Transition: Integrating Health and Mental Health," draft paper, 1979.

3. T. Ben-Dashan, "Case Management: Activities in ESP Strategy States," preliminary report, 1979.

4. P. Caragonne, "Community Maintenance of the Mentally Ill Disabled: A Strategy of Intervention Based Upon a Model of Integrated Services." A report submitted to Mental Health Program Office, Manpower Development Project, Tallahassee, Florida, 1979.

5. P. Caragonne, "Implementation Structures in Community Support Programs: Manpower Implications of Case Management Systems." A report submitted to Mental Health Program Office, Manpower Development Project, Tallahassee, Florida, 1979.

6. Community Support Program, Contract States: Reports, Documents and Proposals, 1977, 1978, 1979.

7. Report of the President from the President's Commission on Mental Health, Vol. I & II, 1978.

8. J.A. Talbott, *The Chronic Mental Patient,* The American Psychiatric Association, Washington, D.C., 1978.

9. J.C. Turner, "Comprehensive Community Support Systems: Definitions, Components and Guiding Principles," NIMH, Rockville, Maryland, 1977.

10. J.C. Turner and C. Kennedy, "The Core Service Agency Concept: Implication for Future Planning and Legislation," working paper, 1979.

11. J.C. Turner and I. Shifren, "Community Support Systems: How Comprehensive?" *New Directions for Mental Health Services,* Vol. 2, 1979.

12. J.C. Turner and W.J. TenHoor, "The NIMH Community Support Program: Pilot Approach to a Needed Social Reform," *Schizophrenia Bulletin,* Vol. 4, No. 3, 1978.

Part II

SYSTEMS/ ORGANIZATIONAL ISSUES

Chapter 4

ORGANIZATIONAL ISSUES
AND CASE MANAGEMENT

Brian Flynn, Ed.D.

Focus of the Presentation

This chapter will focus on the organizational issues affecting and effected by the establishment of case management systems within community mental health centers. It should be noted that organizational issues within and among other types of institutions, particularly state hospitals and other state and community agencies, are equally important. I will focus on community mental health centers since they are one of my major responsibilities in the HEW Region I office and most of my experience is in the community mental health centers.

I have become increasingly interested in and alarmed by the development of a new religion (as opposed to the old religion of the deinstitutionalization) we are calling "case management." Advocates of case management systems are approaching the topic with no less fervor, conviction, and faith than one commonly associates with an intense religious experience. It often appears that to be critical or questioning of case management is, at minimum, unpatriotic and perhaps cruel, inhuman, and callous. In addition, I have become quite concerned regarding the rather gross lack of definitions of what case management is, who should receive management services, and who is responsible for these management activities.

Finally, there are potentially major ramifications for community mental health centers entering into a case management system. These will be described in more detail later. This chapter provides very little in terms of answers to the questions to be raised. In preparing this section it was difficult to identify all of the issues because I'm not really sure what we are talking about when we discuss case management.

What I propose to do is to outline several of the statements that have been made about case management and to explore briefly some of the ramifications, expectations, and issues that arise if one is committed to certain definitions of case management.

Why Is an Organizational Perspective Important?

In general, community mental health centers are just beginning to think in organizational terms. Most centers have gone from being rather small organizations to multi-million dollar corporations with the "assistance" of major federal grants. Centers are just beginning as a whole and fully appreciate the need for being knowledgeable of management systems, organizational diagnosis, etc.

As one who spends a great deal of time in organizational diagnosis activities, I think the organizational chart is of primary importance. It reflects how the organization sees itself and/or how the organization would like others to perceive it. Labels and organizational locations of people and programs reflect status and authority. In addition, the organizational design implies values: who, what is important, what people or programs have most clout and/or value in the organization.

Looking at the organizational structure of a mental health center in terms of case management is critically important because of the necessity of the structure to follow the program rather than vice versa. My experience indicates that many new programs in community mental health centers are established on an organizational chart, and the organizational location is of primary importance in defining the program rather than the program controlling its place on the organizational chart.

For this reason the purpose of this chapter is to examine some of the varying definitions and issues in case management and see how one might expect to see them reflected organizationally. A major goal of this chapter is to avoid the establishment of a case management system and then have the program defined by its organizational location and status.

Statements about Case Management

1. Case management is an advocate for clients in the community.

If one accepts this statement, one might expect to see the case management system closely allied with the consultation/education system in the community mental health system since this is one of the major organizational locations where contact with outside agencies takes place. Second, one might expect to see this rather high in the organizational chart simply because most external operations that have to do with systems integration take place high in the organizational chart rather than low. Third, one might potentially see case management handled by an affiliate organization of the governing board rather than by the main body of the community mental health system.

2. Case management is an advocate for the consumer within the mental health center.

If one defines case management by this statement, it is diagnostic of continuity of care breakdown within the community mental health center. If the client needs an advocate within the system, then something is not working. In addition there is potential overlap between the case management system and the quality assurance program in the mental health center. Finally, one might expect to find unit heads and the division director primarily responsible for case management since this is the organizational location where internal coordination issues are usually handled.

3. Case management is a new service.

If this is the case, then perhaps case management will be established as a separate organizational unit (i.e., a new box on the organizational chart) rather than located within existing programs. A major organizational issue becomes how case management is properly coordinated with other service units when it exists in an independent program unit.

4. Case management is a modality of treatment.

If one sees case management as another modality of treatment (like individual psychotherapy, group treatment, chemotherapy, etc.), then one might expect to see case management function scattered throughout the agency and perhaps not in a separate organizational unit. One might expect to find aspects of case management in, for example, adult outpatient, partial hospitalization, and inpatient services.

5. All clients should have a case manager.

If everyone in the center has a case manager, what then is the difference between a primary therapist and a case manager? Are these roles different? Who is ultimately responsible? Concern is raised regarding the equal competence of all staff to do case management activity. Are the skills different than therapeutic interventions? If so, what are the training needs of case managers?

Financial considerations become increasingly important as more people receive case management. What is the cost to the agency if everyone is involved in case management activities which are currently not paid by third-party reimbursement?

Finally, there is a value judgment made in believing that each person must have a case manager. There is an assumed incompetence in this design that implies that everyone needs case management until he/she proves he/she doesn't. I personally would much rather see a situation where people were assumed not to need case management activities until clinically or environmentally warranted.

6. Only the chronically mentally ill need case management.

If this is believed, it seems most appropriate that there be a close organizational link between after-care, follow-up services, and perhaps partial hospitalization services more than linkage with other programs in the mental health center. Other problems arise in our inability, as a field, to define adequately "chronically ill."

There is a major training issue here. It has been my impression that many clinicians are not adequately trained to deal effectively with the chronically mentally ill. Most clinical training involves primarily exposure to acute types of problems. If one agrees with expanded need for training dealing with the chronically mentally ill, what is the interaction between this need and the continuing education plan for community mental health center staff?

7. The case manager should be your most senior clinician.

In this case one might expect to find the case manager very high in the organizational chart. This is where one finds the most senior clinician in most mental health centers. The question then becomes: Is the best clinician the best prepared individual to provide case management services particularly when these services require skills in dealing with external agencies? Should the senior clinician and the external negotiator be one and the same?

Second, again comes the financial issue. To what extent can the mental health center afford to have its most expensive people provide services that, by and large, are not reimbursable? All centers do this to some extent;

where does one draw the line with providing these types of activities without bankrupting the mental health center? Finally, if the agency's goal is to provide the highest quality service to all clients, is it then not counterproductive to place a disproportionate share of the center's best resources into any one activity or with one client population?

8. Case management need not require clinical training.

If this is the case, then one must find case management rather low in the organizational chart.

What does this mean to negotiations with external systems? Are we asking the case manager to deal from a basically powerless (or limited power) position with people in other agencies who have more status in their organization than the case manager has in his or hers? As a general rule, experience would indicate that negotiations among agencies go best when negotiations take place between peers.

9. Case management is too expensive to mount in a major way.

To make this statement with any type of assurance implies several things within the mental health center. First, it indicates the existence of a management information system that is capable of accounting on an accurate and timely basis the actual cost and revenues produced by its services and clinicians. It implies the ability of the center to cost center case management activities. Finally, it implies the ability of the center to move funds from one program to the other based on varying cost and revenue data.

Overall Concerns

There are several overall concerns that I have regarding case management. I don't believe that these concerns are unresolvable, but I think they must be considered and resolved prior to the establishment of a comprehensive case management system in a community mental health center. These issues are as follows:

(1) Gross lack of definitions in case management. What is case management? Case management for whom? Case management by whom? Case management at what cost?

(2) Is it the community mental health center's mandate to provide "non-mental" types of service (aged housing, jobs, etc.)? I am not saying that the community mental health center has no legitimate role in this area;

however, it is important, particularly for governing boards, to look carefully at what are the varying roles and requirements of community mental health centers. Where does a community mental health center's responsibility stop and another agency's responsibility begin? What is the role of the mental health center in developing non-existent services in the catchment area?

(3) What are the respective roles and responsibilities that the community mental health center and the state mental hospital have with regard to case management? One can assume that most people need case management because of at least two reasons: first, because of clinical necessity; second, by virtue of their dependence on an institutional system. It appears that the state hospital has a major role in the provision of, or assurance of, case management.

(4) Where are the resources to pay for case management? Extreme caution should be exercised by community mental health centers when they contemplate any initiation service without clear indication of where the money is going to come from both to initiate and maintain such a service over time.

(5) To what extent can community mental health centers afford to mount a system of care which involves services that are almost universally currently unreimbursable? All centers do this to some extent. The center needs to consider their long-range financial planning in determining the extent to which they can provide essentially free expanded services.

(6) Centers need to look carefully at different sets of additional resources, cultural factors, and cost factors in delivering case management services to urban, suburban, and rural areas. For example, the necessity for heavy reliance on home visits seems to be an essential part of any case management system. The extent to which that can be provided is very different (programmatically and financially) for urban and rural catchment areas.

(7) What does the implementation of a case management system mean to community mental health centers at different developmental stages and centers of different size? The ability of the community mental health center in its growth stage or early developmental years might be far greater than the ability of an older center faced with declining federal and state funds to mount such a service. It is critically important that the size of the agency and its developmental stage be considered prior to designing and mounting a case management system.

Summary

By these comments I have attempted not to dissuade community mental health centers from mounting case management systems, but to complicate the thinking of center administrators, center staff, and center board members on the issues that need to be considered prior to "jumping on the bandwagon." The benefits to be gained in a case management system in a community mental health center are unquestionable. The establishment of such a system can and will go a long way toward more adequately responding to the needs of the client population addressed by management. We should exercise extreme caution to assure that, when we mount new programs in community mental health centers, the organizational, financial, and value issues are carefully considered.

Chapter 5

CLIENT-BASED PROGRAM ADMINISTRATION

Sharon Miller, M.S.W.

Introduction[1]

The Michigan Department of Mental Health introduced and began funding a function labeled "client services management" in FY 1975/76. Since that time, the function has evolved to include assessment, planning, coordination and facilitation, monitoring, and advocacy responsibilities assumed by the public mental health system. These functional responsibilities are assumed through an administering partnership that includes:

— Individuals seeking, or being ordered to receive, treatment and with whom an "Individual Plan of Service"[2] is developed.
— Individual staff members carrying responsibilities as case administrators/managers. Through the case management process, these staff assure application of quality and continuity of care principles. They also apply the principle of least restrictive treatment suited to individual condition.
— Local program administrators who develop linkage procedures for case managers. These administrators also collect, aggregate, analyze, and use case management information for system development in a specific geographic area.

---

[1]The views expressed throughout this paper are those of the author and do not necessarily reflect official positions of the Michigan Department of Mental Health. The author wishes to acknowledge the efforts of the Office of Services Unification staff toward the development of the paper.

[2]A current "Individual Plan of Service" is required, by policy, for every recipient of public mental health services in Michigan. Case record documentation is currently identified in Department of Mental Health Administration Rules P.A. 258 of 1974, Chapter 7, Rule 7199 (4). Aggregate departmental reporting requirements from the detailed "Individual Plan of Service" are currently undergoing development. See Table 1.

— Central/regional administrators who develop policy guidelines and standards. These administrators use information for monitoring and assessing system performance. They direct and prioritize resource distribution in order to further progress toward system development and management goals.

This four-way administrative partnership reflects multi-level system interdependency in carrying out responsibilities included in the client services management function. Thus individual case managers are maximally effective at coordinating and facilitating activities between agencies, when local program administrators have developed interagency procedures that support staff decisions and bind resources. Likewise, local administrators are maximally effective when central/regional administrators have explored and developed broad policy linkages between state departments with overlapping statutory responsibilities and authorities. Central administrators must also carry out facilitative activities with gubernatorial and legislative agents. The performance interdependency which characterizes the client services management function will be elaborated upon in greater detail following a brief historical review.

Historical Developments[3]

When client services management was introduced in FY 1975/76, the Michigan legislature had expressed a need for improved assessment, planning, coordination, monitoring, and advocacy at the service delivery level. The legislature's specific focus was upon a highly visible but limited number of public mental health clients, i.e., the adult population exiting state institutional facilities but entering alternative community residential programs.

A state level interagency agreement, along with negotiated standards and procedures for guided case administration/management, was introduced to local units as a means of improving direct service delivery. State level planning for implementation of this interagency agreement included a departmental decision to phase-in case management responsibilities for additional population groups over an extended time frame. Ultimately, the

---

[3]Policy guidelines or standards documents referenced in this section are summarized by title and date in Table 2. Copies are available upon request made to the author.

goal was that Community Mental Health (CMH) Boards would assume responsibility for all residents of their geographic catchment area. The boards, under a model system, would develop a uniform system entry and ongoing case management process such that, if a resident entered the public system, the board would plan and monitor the various levels of care and treatment provided until the time of system exit.[4] Entry to and exit from a state facility would be one part of a comprehensive treatment continuum managed by the CMH Board.

Over the next several years, five population groups became specified as target groups for whom CMH boards could assume management responsibilities and thus phase into the complete responsibilities identified in the client services management function. The phase-in, target group approach became formally identified as an option for all CMH boards in the Department's FY 1979/80 Program Policy Guidelines.[5] With this optional approach a board could develop a case management system for adult aftercare (which was mandated) and elect to add responsibility for post-institutionalized children during the subsequent fiscal year. Planned target dates for the specified population groups were required. By 1978, elected levels of responsibility had become identified as indicators of "willingness" consistent with Section 116 (ii) and (g) of the Mental Health Code, Michigan Public Act 258 of 1974. By early 1979, the various statuses of CMH boards with regard to "willingness" and "capacity" for assuming complete responsibility were acknowledged by the Department.

The 1980/81 Program Policy Guidelines invited applications by CMH boards for entering into a special contractual relationship with the Department. Six CMH boards have been accepted as applicants for assuming total responsibility for their residents. An appointed Steering Committee, which includes the applicant CMH Boards, will assist the Department with identifying and developing more specific means of implementation for 1980/81.

The Department has committed resources to assist these CMH boards with building their management capacity over the next year. In addition, the Department will continue to assist CMH boards opting to develop incrementally their capacity. The client services management function is an essential element of building efforts that are underway.

---

[4]A model services arrangement description is provided in Table 3.

[5]The Department issues Program Policy Guidelines on an annual basis. This document guides the planning, program, budgeting process over the 13-18 months preceding the indicated fiscal year.

Capacity Development

Advocacy

Enhancing this component of the client services management function requires assisting clients with participation in and exit from the public mental health system. Every client, professionally evaluated and identified as needing mental health services, must be accorded the right to an "individual plan of service" that identifies his/her program needs, the services that will be provided within available resources, and the case manager that will serve as his/her link to those programs and services in addition to being an assistant in advocating for maximum independence. Within this context, local administrators must develop procedures for staff and clients to advocate based on the "Individual Plan of Service." The procedures will have to support client participation in treatment planning, expanded case record documentation of this participation, as well as consumer representation in the local procedures development process. (See coordination and facilitation component.) Without these local administration developments, advocacy is likely to continue with its base in backup protective systems. Such systems, while valuable as a watchdog function, are primarily rooted in adversarial, investigative, and corrective activities rather than in preventive, meaningful client involvement.

In Michigan, an "Individual Plan of Service" is a legal right only for persons on status with state inpatient facilities. The Department has extended this right to all recipients of public mental health services through policy guidelines and in standards for system entry, case management, and CMH service delivery.

The Department has not, however, assisted implementation through a well-designed approach for training field staff or through building curriculum materials for professional development. It has not been infrequent for this writer to be advised that such participation by clients and/or family members or guardians may be damaging. Such statements appear to indicate a need for building information and educational materials for use by consumer groups and organizations as well as for staff. Finally, the Department may need to require evidence of consumer participation in the annual program planning process as carried out at the local administrative level. At the present time, organizational supports are virtually uncharted at all levels of the public system.

Assessment

While working with clients, case managers perform a variety of needs and service assessment activities. These activities may include:

— Contacting various service providers to assure that pertinent physical, psychological, vocational, educational, cultural, social, economic, legal, environmental, and other factors are appraised for treatment team use in developing a comprehensive "Individual Plan of Service."
— Gathering and providing information to service providers regarding the availability of services and their potential appropriateness for meeting the needs of the client.
— Gathering information related to services identified as needed, but unavailable.
— Consulting with non-mental health service providers to gather information on needs and services as necessary to review and/or update the comprehensive "individual plan of service."

Assessment activities provide a base for planning, coordinating, monitoring, and advocacy for individual clients. Equally important, it is through the case manager's assessment and care record documentation that local administration is assured an information base for need/demand, service accessibility, and service gap assessment. In Michigan, some case managers prepare informational reports regarding the service system and its components. These reports are used for program analysis and evaluation by other administering experts. In some smaller boards these functions are not separately staffed. Irrespective of organizational specialization, however, the "Individual Plan of Service" with its backup case record documentation is *the* baseline from which information for system assessment must be aggregated to carry out higher level administrative activities. Local administrations facilitate case manager effectiveness by developing common in-take processes, unique case number assignments, procedures for case record documentation, and job descriptions that clearly include them as participants in evaluating and planning for development of the local service system. Through these management vehicles, and a participatory philosophy, local administrations become more effective in central/regional administration planning interactions.

State planning requirements are specified annually in the Program Policy Guidelines. The Guidelines usually identify expected sets of analyses and system assessments with regard to state and local policy priorities or program problems. Specified tools, methodologies, and targets of analysis vary as specific program, population, or other priorities change. However, it will become increasingly necessary for all local administrations to provide resources for developing and maintaining "Individual Plans of Service" for all their residents entering the public mental health system. With the increasing expectations for local administration to conduct program analysis, the central and regional staff must increase their capacity to provide technical assistance to them in the areas of evaluation and system assessment. Greater expertise and guidance must be evidenced by producing:

— need/demand assessment tools,
— model program analyses,
— evaluation designs and criteria,
— functional assessment tools,
— training opportunities,
— rewards and incentives for this capacity building effort.

Planning

Case managers carry out planning activities on a daily basis. On a case-by-case basis, a written, comprehensive "Individual Plan of Service" is the product of these efforts. The plan should reflect client or guardian expressions of need, as well as clinical/professional assessments and service availability assessments of mental health and non-mental health providers. It should be developed through a known and administratively supported case planning process. In Michigan, the case planning process is uniformly labeled as the placement review process. The specific placement review procedures vary by geographic area, population group for whom planning must take place, and local administrative preference. However, the State Department of Mental Health issues guidelines specifying minimum participants and product expectations for the local procedures development process.

Needs assessment at entry and placement review decisions are registered for all residents of state facilities. These registrations are aggregated in reports forwarded to CMH boards on a regular basis. Thus, the information can be used for local case management and outreach to individual clients, administrative anticipation of staff needs for placement review participation during an upcoming quarter, and planning for program development. In its 1980/81 Program Policy Guidelines, the Department of Mental Health has required local programs to use supplied needs assessment information to reduce inappropriate placements by 50% during the referenced fiscal year. Community Mental Health planned program revisions developed from the planning information are currently being reviewed and assessed at the central/regional level.

It is the Department's responsibility to "engage in planning for the purpose of identifying, assessing, and enunciating the mental health needs of the state."[6]

State plans expressing regional and inter-regional priorities are expressed in the Department's annual Management Plan which is submitted for inclusion in the Executive Budget. An immediate shortcoming in the Department's ability to enunciate needs through its annual planning, program, and budget process is that many local communities have not chosen to implement a comprehensive entry process with an ongoing case management system so that accurate statistics relating to service demand can be integrated. Consequently, the local planning processes frequently do not reflect the type of client-based data that can be used to support system development. Some consumer group participation may be represented in the local plan submission to the extent that there is representation on the CMH board, ad hoc group utilization, etc. In addition, the state has not issued guidelines or models for needs assessment methodologies in the absence of the preferred client-based system. A major organizational limitation exists with regard to the Department's ability under law to mandate implementation of such a system for operation by CMH boards. Despite the mandate to transfer responsibility to·communities, there are information-sharing restrictions placed upon clinical staff working in community mental health and state components of the system. Thus far, the restrictions have also been extended to demographic information required for planning purposes. CMH boards cannot very well assume responsibility without certain corresponding delegations of authority essential for directing treatment and planning for adequate administration and management of that treatment.

Regional offices were established in 1976 to improve coordinated local CMH and state facility planning. Since that time boards have been required

---

[6]P.A. 258, 1974, Section 116 (f).

to prepare interagency planning strategies with state hospitals as part of their response to the annual Program Policy Guidelines.

These written strategies require identification of local and state agency population group and program element responsibilities over a specified time period. Interagency procedural agreements are to be written in support of the assumed responsibilities. Theoretically, regional director approval indicates coordinated, non-duplicative service planning.

The effectiveness of this organizational adjustment for improved local administration and contribution to the statewide planning effort is still under review. Case studies of local management functions between their planning efforts and subsequent resource development activities are underway.

Coordination and Facilitation

Case managers participate in locally defined and established placement review processes. Through these interagency case planning procedures, the various assessments and service activities completed by mental health and non-mental health providers are coordinated. The procedures are negotiated within state/regional guidelines reflecting state agency policy coordination and clarification of roles, responsibilities, and authority. At the present time local administrators have procedures applicable for adult aftercare service coordination. About half of the new 55 CMH Boards have completed local procedures for the children's aftercare population. Agreements for screening, evaluating, and providing services to unserved or underserved residents of foster case and nursing homes are just being initiated at the local level. Community residents of state facilities are being identified for the 1980/81 fiscal year. Coordination agreements supporting the system entry process will be developed by the pilot contract boards. These local agreements are an essential support for the case manager's daily activities. They assist with issues of authority and resource acquisition for the client.

An extensive inventory of existing state level agreements is being conducted. This inventory will be shared with local administrators. In a departmental review of local agreements completed thus far, there is indication of great variation in substantive content and gaps in policy understanding. Perhaps more significantly the reviews are indicating variations in agreement structure such that many are weak supports for case management staff.

A literature review is assisting departmental staff in preparing an agreement writing guide for local use. This guide will expand upon and better illustrate the generic, essential features of any "agreement." Most mental health personnel at all levels of the system are trained as clinicians and may or may not be educated as case or systems administrators. Both levels of training are needed within local programs.

Coordination and facilitation skills required by case managers are reflected in their daily activities which include:

— Providing immediate facilitation for accessing 24-hour emergency services.
— Maintaining personal contact with clients (and their families) registered for state inpatient services during their episode of care and treatment.
— Providing an up-to-date, complete listing of appropriate mental health resources and explaining how to use these resources to the client.
— Initiating client contact with service providers and when necessary directly assisting the client on an initial visit.
— Maintaining contact with the client and providers as needed to support service provision.
— Providing assistance in applying for non-mental health services recommended in the comprehensive "Individual Plan of Service."
— Determining or facilitating determination of client eligibility for support benefits.
— Developing and providing methods and information to help clients act effectively on their own behalf to obtain benefits.
— Assisting the client in obtaining entitlements when the client is unable or prevented from acting on his own behalf.
— *Consulting* with non-mental health service providers to gather information on needs and services as necessary to review and/or update the comprehensive "Individual Plan of Service."

The department's training program for case managers is underway. In addition, a local state university has expressed interest in preparing graduate curriculum to address the types of strengthened coordinative skills required by case managers.

Monitoring

To the degree that local programs have opted and actually moved to implement a comprehensive system entry and ongoing case management system they have the greatest potential to meet monitoring responsibilities. Case management staff are required to:

— Initiate quarterly reviews of the "Individual Plan of Service" through treatment team conducts or meetings for exchange of information and updating assessments of client need.
— Contact the client through home or program visit at least monthly inquiring as to his/her satisfaction.
— Follow client movement across program components and adjust levels of case management activity in response to the independent functioning ability of the client.
— Record changes in service need and availability, functioning level, and initiate changes in the plan.
— Prepare informational reports for individual case advocacy purposes as well as for use by local administration in system development.

The state department's immediate potential for being knowledgeable about quality and continuity of care is directly related to the level of responsibility assumed by local administrations. Election to assume complete responsibility yields potential for the whole partnership to engage in client-based program administration. Assuming these responsibilities requires building a management information system that captures the decisions and results of the case management process. Without the capacity to collect and aggregate appropriate types and levels of information in an unduplicated manner, local and state/regional administration becomes characterized by weak planning, management, and advocacy. A highly analytical and evaluative capacity becomes essential for assessing system performance against the program budget plan.

In Michigan, the state department is undertaking a major review of its current capacity and identifying potential new information processing models that may assist data-based management.

Interlocking Organizational Considerations

Organizational arrangements for carrying out the client services management function vary greatly. In some instances, the case management staffing is specialized. They are budgeted as administrative staff, and their activities are carried out as a complement to primary therapeutic activities. In other instances, the primary therapeutic staff carry dual responsibilities. Based upon information becoming available from various sites in Michigan and the country, the Department of Mental Health seeks to encourage staff specialized as case managers. This emphasis is valid particularly for clients requiring multiple service delivery following placement from an inpatient facility. Clients receiving only outpatient services, or all services in state inpatient program elements, may be more efficiently and effectively served by having staff with primary therapeutic responsibility carry out the client services management function for their clients. In CMH boards with small service populations this latter, non-specialized model may be the only model possible given staff resources. Life consultation agencies for the developmentally disabled generally include staff responsibility for service activities reportable to the department as part of the client services management function. In all organizational arrangements, case management activities are to be identified and reported separately from direct therapy activities.

To facilitate implementation of the client services management function, at the individual case level, organizational hierarchy and staffing must reflect a number of considerations irrespective of the model utilized:

— Cooperation and communication between treatment staff and specialized case management staff are enhanced by instituting organizational parity between functions and the involved staff.
— In CMH Boards contracting for most or all services, specialized case management staff must be vested with the administrative authority of the Board. However, care must be taken to specify the legitimate activities of "treatment" agencies so that duplication of activity is avoided.
— Recognition of the unique needs of the case management role relative to treatment program functions supports positioning specialized staff within the organization in the manner illustrated in Diagram 1.
— Specialized case management staff require ongoing communication with service delivery staff as well as with non-mental health agencies and staff.
— To facilitate client movement between program elements, the manager needs to communicate with staff from two or more delivery elements simultaneously. This is also a prerequisite for effective coordination of record upkeep, information collection, and quarterly service reviews.

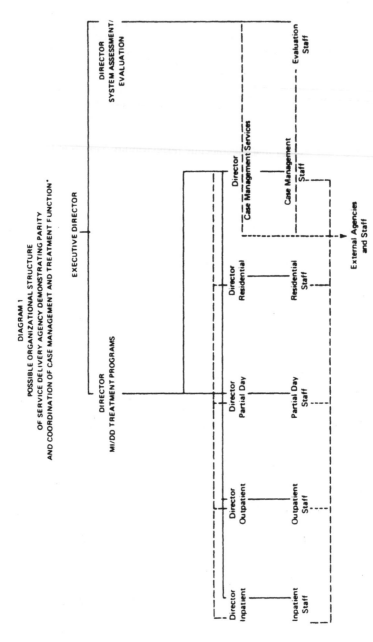

DIAGRAM 1

POSSIBLE ORGANIZATIONAL STRUCTURE
OF SERVICE DELIVERY AGENCY DEMONSTRATING PARITY
AND COORDINATION OF CASE MANAGEMENT AND TREATMENT FUNCTION*

EXECUTIVE DIRECTOR

DIRECTOR
MI/DD TREATMENT PROGRAMS

DIRECTOR
SYSTEM ASSESSMENT/
EVALUATION

Director
Inpatient

Director
Outpatient

Director
Partial Day

Director
Residential

Director
Case Management Services

Inpatient
Staff

Outpatient
Staff

Partial Day
Staff

Residential
Staff

Case Management
Staff

Evaluation
Staff

External Agencies
and Staff

*The author gratefully acknowledges the contributions of Richard Vaughn, Ph.D., Community Support Project, Michigan Department of Mental Health, in preparing this organizational analysis.

— In small boards with only one or a few specialized staff, hierarchical placement should be at the Case Management Services Director, or Director, System Assessment/Evaluation level. This director, however, should be permitted interaction freely at both the staff and supervisory level of the treatment program.

— When the client case management and primary therapeutic staff roles are filled by the same person, it is essential that structural arrangements be made to facilitate discrimination of task responsibility. The supervisory function may be specialized with two individuals performing as treatment supervisor and case management supervisor. This arrangement requires strong administrative support and coordination at the level of the Treatment Program Director.

— All staff assigned responsibilities for the case management function shall be provided training in how to carry out their responsibilities. Such training is additional to whatever other qualifications the individual may have acquired earlier.

As with structural arrangements for case management staff, the local administration's placement of staff responsible for system assessment and evaluation is critical for the multi-level system partnership described at the beginning of this chapter. This impact is especially critical in a CMH board at the point where direct treatment programs are multiple and supervisory staff capacity begins to be added. In Michigan, the critical point appears to be at the CMH board staff level of five to ten positions. Technically specialized expertise for communicating and making decisions on the basis of organized client data assists local executive directors in communicating effectively with their political publics. Relevance upon political finesse, including appeals to meet undocumented "needs" produces short-lived success. The self-described, 18-month turnover rate for executive directors may be one indication of the increasingly greater need for a system of client-based program administration. However, technical expertise, structured and utilized appropriately, is insufficient as a sole solution. Increasingly greater attention should be given at the state level to the statutory base from which the four-level partnership is launched. Each administrative partner requires appropriate tools in order to be accountable for the authority that is vested. Some clarifying observations about requirements for organizational structures in Michigan include:

— Unequal partners cannot positively effect performance. Client authority for participation must be vested in law, and that authority must be applicable at any level and setting of care and treatment provided by the public system.

— The organizational entity accountable for local administration (including case management) and treatment services must be specified.

— Resources for demonstrating accountability must be vested at the administrative level specified as accountable. Essential resources include:

— Authority over treatment processes such as authorizing and registering the treatment plan, purchasing services (including from state hospitals), monitoring service provisions, and standards compliance.

— Information collection, aggregation, and processing capacity across public system providers.

— Budgetary allocations directly to the accountable entity such that cost-effective and efficient trade-offs can be achieved.

— Billing and expenditure control capacity.

— The central administration's authority and responsibility for statewide system performance must be distinguished from local administrative and essential resources (as noted above) correspondingly authorized.

Table 1

Department of Mental Health Administrative Rules to PA 258
Chapter 7, Rule 7199 (4)

An individualized plan of service shall contain, whenever applicable:

(a) A statement of the nature of specific problems or disabilities and specific needs.

(b) Evaluation of strengths as well as weaknesses.

(c) Evaluation of the degree of physical disability and the plan for remedial or restorative measures.

(d) Evaluation of the degree of mental disability and the service plan for appropriate measures to be taken to relieve treatable conditions and distress and to compensate for non-reversible impairment.

(e) Evaluation of capacity for social interaction and plan for appropriate measures to increase adaptive capacity.

(f) Evaluation of environmental and physical limits required to safeguard health and safety.

Table 1 (*continued*)

(g) Determination of the least restrictive treatment or habilitation setting necessary to achieve the purposes of admission.

(h) A statement of and rationale for intermediate and long-range goals, specifying the manner in which the facility can improve the resident's condition with a projected timetable for attainment.

(i) Proposed staff involvement with the resident in order to attain goals, including a minimum number of individual contacts and consultations planned between the resident and professional staff, the expected minimum number of hours of the consultations in each 30-day period.

(j) The frequency and extent of physical examinations.

(k) Criteria to be met for release or discharge, and prognosis for placement.

(l) Notation of therapeutic tasks, labor, personal housekeeping, recreation, or other scheduled activities to be performed, including those as a condition of residence in a small group living arrangement and a rationale for these in relation to goals.

(m) An estimated date for release or discharge with a proposed date for development of a plan of service needed after release or discharge, including participation of community mental health services.

(n) Drug regimens by type, dosage, and frequency; changes in medication or dosages; and notation of effects and behavior changes.

(o) Dates for reviews at intervals not less than every 90 days and by whom the review shall be done, including provision for a written assessment of progress toward goals and reasons for progress or lack of progress.

(p) Documentation of a restriction or limitation of rights and any restraint or seclusion.

(q) Record of surgery; electro-convulsive therapy or other procedures intended to produce convulsions or coma; experimental procedures; family planning services, including sterilization and abortion; guardianships; legal and other protective services.

Table 2

Policy Guidelines and Standards Documents

1. Memorandum to All Community Mental Health Board Directors and All State Hospital and Facility Directors from Donald C. Smith, M.D. *Subject:* Client Services Management - A Departmental Policy and Procedural Framework for Adult Community Placement, Residential, and Aftercare Services. January 27, 1976.
2. Memorandum of Agreement between Michigan Department of Mental Health and the Michigan Department of Social Services on the Adult Community Placement Services Process for Mental Health Clients. September 3, 1975.
3. Memorandum to All Hospital and Facility Directors and All Community Mental Health Services Boards from Donald C. Smith, M.D. *Subject:* Revision of the Working Guidelines for Placement Review Committees - Phase I. May 9, 1977.
4. Interagency Statement on Coordination of Services for Children Returning to Communities from State Mental Health Facilities. September 25, 1978. Standards and Criteria for Case Planning and Service Assurance to Children Exiting State Mental Health Facilities. Revised December 1978.
5. Interagency Agreement on Screening, Referral, and Mental Health Evaluation of Adults Placed in Alternative Care Settings Prior to January 1976 by Michigan Department of Mental Health, Michigan Department of Public Health and Michigan Department of Social Services. April 1979.
6. Draft Standards for System Entry and Ongoing Client Services Management. January 1979.
7. Michigan Department of Mental Health, Inpatient Needs Assessment and Case Registration Manual. December 1978.
8. Fourth Annual Program Policy Guidelines, Fiscal Year 1980–81. Michigan Department of Mental Health. May 1979.

Table 3

Model Client Services Array

This chart displays a model array of mental health system services. It provides a single source for information about and access to services. The model eliminates the confusing and inefficient duplication of access points and services that exists in the state's current system. The model does *not* show the organization or units which would provide services.

Information about mental health services is provided to the general public and to agencies that are likely to have contact with people who need mental health services. The potential mental health client and others who are interested in his or her well-being may then request services, either directly or indirectly by referral from another agency. The request may be either voluntary or involuntary, through court action. Following the request for mental health services, the potential client's functioning and services needs are diagnosed and assessed.

If, after assessment, the person is determined inappropriate for mental health services, either no services are provided or the person is referred back to another agency that can better meet his or her needs. If mental health services are appropriate, one or more of those services are provided, sometimes in combination with the services of non-mental health agencies.

Following a period of service delivery, the client's progress is evaluated. Evaluation findings may result in either: the provision of further mental health services, service termination, or referral for services from a non-mental health agency.

(Table 3 continued on next page)

Table 3 (continued)

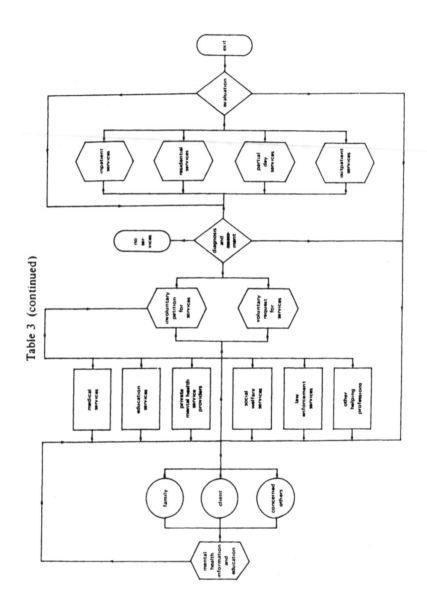

Part III

LEGAL/ETHICAL ISSUES

Chapter 6

CLIENTS' RIGHTS
IN A CASE MANAGEMENT SYSTEM

David Wolowitz, J.D.

A number of successful lawsuits throughout the nation have propelled the recent trend toward deinstitutionalization of the mentally ill and mentally retarded.[1] This trend toward deinstitutionalization appears to be a primary motivation for the development of a case management system. A case management system is designed to insure that individuals released from institutions receive appropriate supportive services to enable them to remain in their own communities.

One of the purposes of a case management system is to enhance the rights of the disabled by keeping them in the community and out of institutions. However, the provision of services that maintain clients outside of institutions does not insure the protection of client interests.

There is, I believe, a correlation between an increase in social services and a decrease in the autonomy of clients dependent on those services. Much of the history of the development of social services has involved recipients yielding to the discretionary authority of service providers in return for receiving services. In recounting the rise of social services in the United States, one commentator provides the following analysis:

> Liberal society, which is to say caring society, came mostly to believe that the only difficulty with social services was that there weren't enough to go around; the public sector they argued, was being starved in the midst of private affluence. If the quality of public education, public housing, child care, medical care, and welfare was not what it should be, it was primarily because of inadequate resources. What was needed, according to the liberals, was more, not less, public intervention.
>
> This undifferentiated view of social services, and the political context in which the struggle to provide social services took place,

tended to blind liberals to certain unintended consequences of their good works. Because their motives were benevolent, their ends good, and their purpose caring, *they assumed the posture of parents* toward the receipt of their largesse. They failed utterly to resist the impulse toward paternalism, which in another context Bernard Bailyn called "the endlessly propulsive tendency" of power to expand itself and to establish *dominion* over people's lives. They eagerly embraced such dominion and persuaded themselves that by doing so they were helping the helpless. Dominion became legitimate: those who managed social services—not infrequently liberals themselves—came to enjoy a degree of discretionary power over their clients that normally only parents are allowed over their children. As a result, they infantilized those they intended to help, and denied them their rights.[2]

My concern, and the focus of this chapter, is to minimize the loss of autonomy for clients in a case management system. Recipients of supportive services should not have to foresake legal rights or human dignity as the price of the services. A case management system should be designed to maintain, to the fullest extent possible, the clients' control over their lives while permitting them opportunities to utilize available services.

Although there are a number of legal issues raised by a case management system, I will discuss three in particular: avoiding conflict of interest, protecting privacy, and safeguarding confidentiality. For analytical purposes, I have broken down the case management system into what appears to be its three basic functions: advocacy on behalf of clients, coordination (including planning, referral, and evaluation), and treatment. The legal issues apply equally to each function, but for the sake of brevity I have chosen to relate each function to a particular legal issue.

Client Advocacy and Potential Conflict of Interest

One proposed role for case managers is to act on behalf of clients to remedy problems with other agencies that provide services to the same clients. This is the so-called "advocacy" role for case managers. Unlike lawyers, lay advocates are not bound by the Code of Professional Responsibility which prohibits conflicts of interest for attorneys.[3] I am deeply concerned that case managers will be unable to overcome real or potential conflicts of interest that interfere with zealous advocacy on behalf of their clients.

Most of the services to the mentally and developmentally disabled are provided by the state, either directly through state agencies or indirectly through programs funded by the state. When problems arise relating to services or assistance to disabled clients, a case manager must be prepared to confront representatives of the state. Case managers themselves employed by the state have an obvious conflict of interest when they have to advocate on behalf of a client against their employer. In addition to the natural instinct for preservation of one's job, employees tend to identify with the interests of their employer. State employees are no exception.[4]

One possible solution to this obvious conflict of interest is to make the case management system part of an independent state developmental disabilities advocacy agency.[5] An agency created by statute would have the authority to pursue legal remedies and the statute could be drawn to provide independence from other state agencies.[6] However, the staff of such an agency may not be prepared or willing to serve the coordination and treatment functions of a case management system.

A case management system administered by a private agency would have a less obvious conflict of interest with the state. The extent of the agency's reliance on state funding will be an important factor in determining the extent of the potential conflict of interest. Additionally, even if the overall percentage of state funding is relatively small, the perception of the agency's management as to the security of its funding is crucial. If agency administrators believe that state funding, at whatever level, may be easily jeopardized, the staff will be under pressure to avoid conflicts with the state.

To minimize conflict of interest between an agency receiving state funding and its clients, funding contracts should be long-term and carefully drawn to prevent arbitrary revocation of funding. The purpose and consequences of the advocacy role should be understood and acknowledged by both the agency and the state prior to implementing the advocacy system. Realistically, an agency receiving state funding for a case management system must expect that a zealous advocacy program is likely to endanger its funding. Therefore, the surest way to avoid conflict of interest is to drop the advocacy role from the case management program and refer clients in need of such assistance to other, more independent, advocacy groups.

Coordination of Client Services and the Right to Privacy

Another function for case managers is coordinating the various services available to their clients. Coordination requires the sharing of information about clients. We live in an information-oriented society. Information in the possession of government and private agencies, in files and in computers, has a way of taking on exaggerated importance. Although the sharing of certain information may be useful and necessary, the sharing of all information is, at best, a waste of time and, at worst, harmful.[7]

Each of us has a fundamental right of personal privacy which the United States Supreme Court has elevated to a constitutional principle.[8] This right of privacy is not forfeit if one is mentally or otherwise disabled.

A case manager's efforts to coordinate client services must be tempered by a respect for the client's right to privacy. When disclosing information to third parties, three important principles should apply. First, no information should be released without the informed consent of the client or the client's legal representative. Second, only the minimum information necessary to achieve the desired purpose should be released, and only to the appropriate parties. Third, recipients of information should not be permitted to share the information with other agencies or persons.

The third principle is likely to be the most difficult to implement. With the advent of electronic data processing, efforts to control the spread of information have become increasingly frustrating.[9] A 1977 report on therapeutic confidentiality focused on the special problems caused by electronic data processing.

> Significant confidentiality issues are raised when electronic data processing involves accumulation of client-identified data outside the facilities where care and treatment are being provided. First, there is the proliferation of client-identifiable information to two previously nonexistent sources—the "outside" computer facility and the transmission lines—from which confidential information can be leaked. A second serious concern arises when a single computer facility receives client-identified information from a number of mental health facilities. Such data banks represent a reservoir of mental health information removed from the mental health services provider, and a remote source of information is more susceptible to misinterpretation or misuse than the original source.
>
> Third, data banks contain a great volume of information that could injure, embarrass or discredit individuals. Obviously, all compilations of such records, including paper files at mental health facilities, have the same potential. But when confidential information is amassed from several facilities on a county-region- or state-wide basis and is computerized, a much more inviting target is created.
>
> The particular characteristics which render data banks such a unique hazard to confidentiality and privacy are the volume of data

they contain, the speed with which they can be surveyed and the small number of people who need to be corrupted to obtain the data. By contrast, improper attempts to gain confidential information through individual facilities are much less efficient and much more risky.[10]

The report goes on to propose legislation to safeguard information in electronic data processing systems.[11] Without legislative and procedural safeguards, it may be impossible for a case management system to store and share information necessary to the coordination of client services without significantly jeopardizing the privacy of the very clients it is attempting to serve.

In addition to an individual's constitutionally protected right to avoid disclosure of personal information, the right of privacy includes an individual's interest in making important personal decisions free from state interference.[12] Participation in a case management system should not be at the expense of personal autonomy. Unfortunately, the term "case management" itself suggests loss of control by the client. Individuals are depersonalized by referring to them as "cases," not clients. The term further suggests that these "cases" are so helpless that they must be "managed," not merely assisted. Although the term "case management" may, in fact, be harmless academic or administrative jargon,[13] it may be offensive to potential clients and to client organizations.[14]

Case managers should avoid the popular prejudice that the mentally and developmentally disabled are all incompetent. For example, mental illness must not be confused with incompetency. "It is clear that mental illness is not the equivalent of incompetency, which renders one incapable of giving informed consent to medical treatment."[15] Individuals not adjudicated incompetent retain all of their rights to make decisions controlling their lives.[16]

Even clients adjudicated incompetent are not necessarily totally incapable of participating in decisions about their lives. Increasingly, the concept of limited guardianship is being applied in incompetency proceedings.[17] Case managers cannot substitute their judgment for clients who have guardians; only the guardian has the final say in decisions about the ward.

All clients retain certain fundamental rights despite their disability.[18] A case management system should respect the rights of its clients to privacy and freedom of choice. Clients must not be coerced to participate in a case management system. Receipt of state services should not be dependent on participation. Grievance procedures should be established, publicized, and enforced for those clients who do participate.

Treatment and the Threat to Confidentiality

A third function proposed for case managers is the establishment of a therapeutic relationship with their clients. Presumably clients will receive their primary treatment from professionals outside the case management system. The case manager's role will be to supplement and enhance treatment provided by others. Much of the treatment provided by outside professionals and case managers will relate to psychiatric problems and most clients will be involved in some form of psychotherapy.

Most mental health professionals perceive confidentiality to be a prerequisite for the free and open communication essential to effective therapy. "Unless a patient . . . is assured that . . . information (revealed by him) can and will be held in the utmost confidence, he will be reluctant to make the full disclosure upon which diagnosis and treatment . . . depends."[19] Client communications to a case manager will not automatically be privileged. A case management system that is not carefully designed may even result in the destruction of the client's privilege with other mental health professionals.

Generally, communications between a patient and a mental health professional are privileged only when covered directly[20] or indirectly[21] by a specific statute.[22] Therefore, communications made by a client to a case management professional not covered by a confidentiality statute will not be privileged. To make matters worse, revelation of otherwise privileged communications to a third party not covered by a privilege generally destroys the privilege.[23] Thus a client who shares treatment information with a case manager not covered by a confidentiality statute may be waiving the protective privilege.

To protect its client's right to confidentiality, the case management system should be designed either to omit the treatment function altogether or to bring client communications under the protection of a confidentiality statute. Legally, the simplest way to insure confidentiality is to enact a statute specifically protecting communications to case managers.[24] Realistically, legislatures are reluctant to create new privileges. Without a statute that specifically applies to case managers, steps must be taken to hire case managers already covered by the provisions of existing statutes. This may prove to be difficult as most statutes cover only professionals who are unlikely to be employed as case managers, such as physicians and certified psychologists. Few states have social worker confidentiality statutes, although the number is increasing. Alternatively, confidentiality might be protected if the case management treatment function was an arm of a community mental health center or other treatment oriented agency, depending on the laws of the jurisdiction.

Even if the problem of creating a privilege in a case management setting is overcome, a case management system must further be designed to protect and maintain the privilege. The privilege, it should be remembered, belongs to the client, not the case manager.[25] The case manager is therefore bound by the decisions of the client or his legal representative relating to release of information. Valid authorization to release privileged information requires the informed consent of the client. Informed consent requires that the client know what information is being released, the purpose of the release, and the identity of the recipient. Thus informed consent requires client access to his or her records containing the information to be released.

A case management therefore must be designed to permit reasonable client access to their own records. The federal government and many states already have statutes permitting patient access to their treatment records.[26] However, there is vehement opposition in the treatment community to client access to psychiatric and psychological records. Despite this opposition, the Privacy Protection Study Commission and others strongly support client access rights to their records.[27]

Creative solutions to the problem of client access to records have been suggested, including a proposed dual record keeping system endorsed by such diverse groups as the American Society of Internal Medicine, the American Civil Liberties Union, and the IBM Medical Department.[28] Although the problem is difficult, it is one which a case management system must confront and resolve in order to protect the rights of its clients.

Conclusion

A case management system is a new variation on an old theme. It is an attempt by professionals and experts to help people whom they perceive to be in need of their assistance. Undoubtedly the architects of the system sincerely believe that they are acting in the best interests of the proposed clients. Yet the system has obvious potential for violating the rights of its disabled clients.

There is a certain irony that the case management system is a response to court victories for clients' rights. Advocates of case management should not deceive themselves or others into believing that a system promoting the deinstitutionalization of the disabled inevitably promotes the interests of the disabled. The rights of the disabled historically have been ignored and trampled in institutions. The same injustices could easily continue in the community.

The purpose of this chapter has been to demonstrate the many potential legal pitfalls of a case management system. A successful case management system ought to strive continually to enable clients to control their own lives to the fullest extent possible. Participants in a case management system must acknowledge the rights of the disabled clients. Only if there is respect for the rights of the disabled clients will client autonomy be truly enhanced. The fundamental issue for a case management system is client self-determination, because after all is said and done no one knows and understands the needs and interests of the disabled better than the disabled themselves.

NOTES

1. *Wyatt v. Stickney*, 344 F. Supp. 373 (M.D.Ala. 1972), aff'd, 503 F.2d 1305 (5th Cir. 1974), *O'Connor v. Donaldson*, 422 U.S. 563 (1975), *Halderman v. Pennhurst*, 46 U.S.L.W. 1113 (E.D.Pa. 1/31/78), *Wuori v. Zitnay*, 2 MDLR 693 (D.Me. 7/14/78).

2. P. 107, Glasser, Ira, "Prisoners of Benevolence: Power Versus Liberty in the Welfare State," in Gaylin, *Doing Good, The Limits of Benevolence* (1978).

3. Canon 5 of the Code of Professional Responsibility states: "A lawyer should exercise independent professional judgment on behalf of a client." Ethical consideration EC 5-1 states: "The professional judgment of a lawyer should be exercised, within the bounds of the law, solely for the benefit of his client and free of compromising influences and loyalties. Neither his personal interests, the interests of other clients, nor the desires of third persons should be permitted to dilute his loyalty to his client."

4. In a decision of an appeal by two recipients of Aid to Families with Dependent Children (AFDC) claiming unfair treatment by the New Hampshire Division of Welfare dated December 21, 1978, Edward P. Pound, Welfare Hearing Officer for the State of New Hampshire ruled as follows:

> The evidence is not conclusive as to whether these clients may have been unfairly treated. There has, however, been a pattern of cases involving the allegations of clients as to the nature of their treatment by the District Office . . .

> In the last two years, there have been at least some five hearings involving the complaint that the District Office had, in one way or another, failed to recognize the right of a recipient. With the exception of one case there was some evidence to support these complaints. This pattern does lend further weight to the existing complaints of these appellants that they were not treated fairly by the District Office.

> The Hearings Officer takes note that there is evidence to support a finding that the appellants did not receive full, fair, and equitable treatment to which they were entitled.

5. Such an agency is mandated by the Developmental Disabilities Assistance and Bill of Rights Act, Pub.L. 94-103, 42 U.S.C. §6001-6081 (Suppl. V 1975) which requires that states create a protection and advocacy system by October 1, 1977 to qualify for federal funds for developmental disabilities programs.

6. See, e.g., "Model Statute for Establishing a Developmental Disabilities Advocacy Agency" 2 MDLR 767-793 (May-June 1978).

7. See, e.g., Levine, Carol, "Sharing Secrets: Health Records and Health Hazards," in *Hastings Center Report*, pp. 13-15, (December, 1977).

8. *Griswold v. Connecticut*, 381 U.S. 479 (1965), *Roe v. Wade*, 410 U.S. 113 (1973), *Moore v. City of East Cleveland*, 431 U.S. 494 (1977).

9. See, e.g., Schmeck, Harold M., Jr., "The Easy Access To Medical Records," *N.Y. Times* (March 6, 1977).

10. "Legal Issues in State Mental Health Care: Proposals for Change, Therapeutic Confidentiality," 2 Mental Disability Law Reporter, 337-354 (September-December, 1977).

11. The report (see note 10) includes the following statutory proposal:

Electronic Data Processing by Mental Health Facilities.

(a) No confidential information with client identifiers shall be recorded on electronic data processing equipment outside a mental health facility by any governmental body, branch, or agency, except upon the voluntary and informed authorization of the client in accordance with this act. No person shall be denied treatment for refusing to grant such authorization.

(b) Confidential information regarding current clients may be recorded on electronic data processing equipment outside a mental health facility only if (i) all client identifiers remain at the treating facility; (ii) the client identifiers are delivered, within 60 days after a client ceases to participate in diagnosis or treatment, to a person or persons under the direct supervision of the director of the treating facility, which person or persons are denied access to the electronic data processing equipment and are responsible for the safekeeping of the client identifiers pursuant to this act.

(c) The client identifiers may be released by the persons specified in subsection (b) (ii) for purposes of reactivating access to confidential information stored on electronic data processing equipment when, and only when, (i) the client to whom such information pertains has reentered diagnosis or treatment at such facility; (ii) a request for confidential information which may be honored under the provisions of this act has been received; (iii) it is necessary for auditors regularly employed by the state to inspect electronic data equipment to ensure strict and complete compliance with this act, *provided that* such inspections shall not involve the removal of such encoding means and devices, or copies or other reproductions thereof from a mental health facility; (iv) confidential information is required for a fair hearing in connection with the dismissal of an employee charged with violating this act; or (v) it is necessary for use in a civil or criminal action arising out of violations of this act.

(d) No later than three years after a client has ceased to participate in diagnosis or treatment at a facility, either the client identifiers shall be destroyed or all electronically processed data pertaining to such client shall be returned to data processing personnel at such facility.

12. *Roe v. Wade*, 410 U.S. 113 (1973), *Whalen v. Roe*, 429 U.S. 589 (1977), *Carey v. Population Services Inter.*, 431 U.S. 678 (1977). See, generally, Henkin, "Privacy and Autonomy," 74 Colum. L. Rev. 1410 (1974).

13. Jargon is no stranger to case management proposals. Consider, for example, the following paragraph from a chapter on "Service Process" in an article describing the case management system by Ron Gerhard:

Case managers maintain continuous relationships with consumers, assisting, whenever required, in the alleviation of crisis-provoking situations. They also convene planning-linking conferences at every major decision point throughout the individual's stay in the service system. These conferences are attended by the consumer, significant others from the consumer's folk-support system, and those service providers with specific knowledge of the consumer and/or the service alternatives under consideration. All major service decisions are made at these conferences.

14. See, generally, *Advocacy Now: The Journal of Patient Rights and Mental Health Advocacy* (May 1979). See also Severo, "Mental Patients Seek 'Liberation' in Rising Challenge to Therapies," *N.Y. Times*, p. A1 (December 11, 1978).

15. *Scott v. Plante*, 532 F.2d 939 (3rd Cir. 1976); *Rennie v. Klein*, C.A. No. 77-2624 (D.N.J. December 9, 1978).

16. See, e.g., N.H. RSA 135-B:42, *Rights of Patients*. The patient's right to individual dignity shall be respected at all times and upon all occasions including any occasion when the patient is taken into custody, treated, detained, or transported pursuant to this chapter or any other chapter relating to mental health. No person who is receiving treatment for mental illness shall be deprived of any legal rights; provided, however, that if such a person has been adjudicated as incompetent, his rights may be limited to the same extent as the rights of any incompetent person are limited at general law. See, generally, Plotkin, "Limiting the Therapeutic Orgy: Mental Patients' Right to Refuse Treatment," 72 Nw.U.L.Rev. 461 (1977).

17. See, generally, Horstman, Peter M., "Protective Services For the Elderly: The Limits of Parens Patriae," 40 Mo.L.Rev. 215 (Spring 1975).

18. *Karmowitz v. Department of Mental Health*, Civ. No. 73-19434 (Cir. Ct. Wayne County, Mi., 7/10/73) reprinted in Miller, *The Mental Health Process* 567 (1976), *Rennie v. Klein*, supra.

19. Senate Committee on the Judiciary, comments on Evidence Code, §1014, cited in *Tarasoff v. Regents*, 529 P.2d 553 (Cal. 1974).

20. E.g., NH RSA 329:26. Doctor-Patient Privilege: "The confidential relations and communications between a physician or surgeon licensed under provisions of this chapter and his patient are based on the same basis as those provided by law between attorney and client, and except as otherwise provided by law, no such physician or surgeon shall be required to disclose such privileged communications."

21. E.g., July 1, 1979 amendment to N.H. RSA 329:26: Confidential relations and communications between a patient and any person working under the supervision of a physician or surgeon that are customary and necessary for diagnosis and treatment are privileged to the same extent as though those relations or communications were with such supervising doctor or surgeon.

22. But the Pennsylvania Supreme Court recently found a non-statutory right to confidentiality for a patient in psychotherapy based on the patient's fundamental right of privacy. *In re "B," Appeal of Dr. Loren Roth*, No. 150 (Penn. 10/5/78).

23. Cleary, *McCormick on Evidence*, p. 216 (1972).

24. See, e.g., N.H. RSA 167:30 Confidential Character of Public Assistance Records and N.H. RSA 167:31 Misuse of Lists and Records.

25. Cleary, *McCormick on Evidence*, p. 192 (1972).

26. For a state by state summary, see Auerbach, Melissa, *Getting Yours: A Consumer Guide to Obtaining Your Medical Records*, Health Research Group (July 1978).

27. *Personal Privacy in an Information Society: The Report of the Privacy Protection Study Commission*, U.S. Government Printing Office (July 1977), "How To Reduce Patients' Anxiety: Show Them Their Hospital Records," Medical World News (1/13/75); Shenkin, B., "Giving the Patient His Medical Record: A Proposal to Improve the System," 289 New England Journal of Medicine 688 (9/27/73).

28. Westin, Alan F., "Medical Records: Should Patients Have Access? A Proposal For Dual Record Keeping," Hastings Center Report, pp. 23-28 (December 1977).

Chapter 7

ETHICS OF CASE MANAGEMENT

Henry E. Payson, M.D.

We have been talking about care or the management of care of people, who have been, and still are, severely ill or mentally retarded. As David Wolowitz points out, there seems to be an inevitable danger of loss of privacy and confidentiality (as well as bureaucratization of the managers themselves). This might endanger rather than protect client's rights because these rights are sometimes (if not often) in conflict with the organizational interest of service agencies. For example, a welfare office is ordered to reduce welfare expenditures. Welfare workers would then not win the boss' appreciation for encouraging eligible clients to apply for full benefits. A client's rights might even be in conflict with the case manager's personal and professional interest. The less restriction and greater freedom of a client, the more community exposure to deviant behavior reactions could jeopardize the manager's job and personal security. Case managers would be government employees. How frequently have we encountered public servants who will protect a client's rights as vigorously as their own? Every positive example is rare enough to inspire us all.

Nevertheless, the complexity and variety of services which deinstitutionalized citizen needs will require comprehensive planning, coordination, and red-tape cutting for proper community management. It hardly needs to be said that failure of community management of persons with mental retardation and mental illness would make more restrictive reinstitutionalization unavoidable in the future.

If the case manager is not really a creature of cynical imagination (a Byzantine device to deflect civil rights litigation away from commissions, directors, and supervisors?) and if the state honestly seeks more effective individualized forms of management of deinstitutionalized care, the need for case managers is great, indeed. All of us working for better mental health and mental retardation services would want such case management to be successful. However, I fear that it might be impossible. There are formidable problems.

One problem is that the tasks encountered in management of chronic disability will always be multiple and compounded. No task can be isolated and dealt with independently, so that it is almost certain that successful outcome will be impossible to assess. Evaluations of management of multiple tasks will be testimonial and non-objective at worst, and equivocal at best. As I will point out, the utility of such management will be comparable to that of physicians prior to the 19th century.

Another problem is that even powerful government leaders fail to make public services effective and satisfactory, even when motivated by huge political stakes. How can a case manager drawing a fixed salary, let alone be motivated, much less succeed without authority to force compliance by other governmental workers? In a state such as New Hampshire, where budgets of every department (as well as that of the case managers) will always be lean if not under-funded, how can case managers alternatively obtain and pay for services from the private sector? Will the legislature make more funds available for the disabled than for highways, schools, and police functions? Case management is not merely knowing where the services are and how to obtain them for a client. There are problems of agency territoriality, and the successful case worker must know how to manage such informal but formidable vectors such as seniority, obligation, favoritism, and *quid pro quo*. Successful manipulation of these *and* private resources will require a consummate politician. Would not one so miscast as to be a successful case manager make a better governor? Senator? Power is the ability to influence and bring the behavior of others into a cooperative effort towards long-range goals. The case manager will start his/her work with very little power over anyone other than his/her client.

The case manager is badly needed, nonetheless. How can case management get done? I think that the history of medical ethics suggests a possible and maybe even practical approach. The case manager's role that I have described compares to that of physicians prior to the advent of anesthesia and antisepsis in the mid-19th century. The pre-19th-century physician had, with rare exceptions, no political or governmental power. His treatments were of equivocal benefit, and yet he was responsible for the protection and optimal treatment of his patients. Clinical failure was frequent, and he was the most accessible target for blame when anything went wrong. Yet, the healing profession has always survived and has been recognizably as comfortable and secure as any other skilled trade. For more than 1500 years physicians have been sought and assigned case management. How have they survived failure without power? There has always been great utility in comfort, competence, loyalty, and protection, but medicine has never had monopoly of such services. Is there an historical explanation of the survival value of the physician image/role? I think there is, and that it can still be used for the survival of non-physician case managers who will be powerless but, nonetheless, responsible for care services to severely disabled persons. I want to suggest that the ethical creed of physicians has not only inspired the most tolerable professional behavior, but has accomplished the most successful ancient public relations feat of all time. It has maintained an agreeable image of the physician in the public mind. The image and the behavior have also created a special power and influence which has facilitated the healing role. It should be added that when all treatment effort failed the image also left the physician with a personal security which favored his personal survival.

Ethics are usually thought of as a broad field of philosophic considerations focused mainly on moral good and social obligations. Over the past 2400 years such concepts and values have undergone continuous evolution and sometimes radical change. In contrast, *medical* ethics have been highly traditioned and little changed. Although they appear to have originated in the philosophy of the Pythagorean school,[1] there was gradual but permanent acceptance of Hippocratic ideals. Rather than being expressions of moral justice or deontological or teleological concepts of social or spiritual good, the Hippocratic Corpus is a practical handbook of how-to-do, as well as a public enunciation of professional deportment. The unchanging qualities of the credo of deportment seem to be its own great secret of survival and of the survival of physicians who were wise enough to adopt it.

The Hippocratic Oath was a combination of covenant and oath: a covenant binding the physician to the professional family of doctors and a public promise to practice solely for the well-being of patients, to abstain from all injury and exploitation, to guard all confidences, and to live a pure and holy life. In the entire Hippocratic Corpus there is no explanatory justification for such deportment. Most probably this is because it was the model of Pythagorean deportment at the time of the peak of the system's importance in the fourth century B.C. As I have just said, the adoption by non-Pythagoreans after the system began its political decline was, in part, a ref-

---

[1]The Hippocratic School was part of a Pythagorean Society and was not representative of customary healing practice in Ancient Greece. Pythagoreans were natural food fadists and abstemious clean-life advocates whose notion of purity, holiness, and avoidance of role ambiguity is expressed in the Hippocratic Oath. The refusal to assist a suicide (euthanasia), to perform abortions, and to remove bladder stones was exceptional to ancient practice, and there was exploitation of confidence and weakness. Some writers believe the oath itself was a reaction against practices prevalent around 400 B.C.

uge and in part a reaction against the then prevalent abuses that the Oath interdicted. The Hippocratic non-Pythagoreans were a small minority of practitioners before the rise of Christian doctrines which may not have been entirely coincidental.[2]

Care of the very sick has always been dangerous. In Hellenistic times there was no civil recourse to damage suits for professional negligence or failure. A beaten or dead physician was regarded as no irreparable loss. Although it may not be difficult to visualize the almost total lack of community protection of the individual in ancient times, it is hard to appreciate the effect of manners and deportment upon personal security when passions were aroused by death and suffering.

When threatened by possible loss of life or limb, it seems to be a characteristic human reaction to submit to anyone believed to have healing powers. But assumption of the patient or sufferer's role is regressive, dependent, and child-like. The role has a rationale: "If he can make me better I must submit to him and obey for he can make me worse." The power to cure can surely kill. Hope of survival embellishes the healer with magical expectation. But the process of submission also simultaneously provokes and suppresses rage as well as relinquishes personal responsibility. The patient and family then tend to blame the physician for unfavorable results. The ethics of the physician as promulgated in the Hippocratic Corpus boil down to this:

1. Make the patient's relatives assume a maximum responsibility for every failure to trust and obey the prescriptive orders of the physician.
2. Make God or Nature responsible by pessimistic prognostications (to the relatives) before the treatment begins.
3. Maintain an image of unselfish dedication, loyalty, piety, and immaculate deportment which reduces the possibilities of becoming a scapegoat when all efforts fail.
4. Avoid all conflicts of interest which might involve political power, blackmail, sexual advantage and forsake all license to handicap or kill.
5. Treat all as brothers regardless of political persuasion. In other words, uphold the laws and justice, but remain apolitical.

---

[2]For some written comment on the coincidence of Pythagorean doctrine with Jewish (Essenian) and Christian teachings, see Dolger Antike U. Christentum ref. Edelstein L. IV 1934.

These principles appear to have been the principles of medical survival. In order to avoid retaliation for failure, the physician avoided assumption of all but the purely healing powers. The public was to be encouraged to believe that every physician is as committed to the total restraint of exploitation or temptation. Any other form of power, other than healing power, would identify points of possible conflicts of interest and personal hazards. For survival of the modern case manager, ancient medical deportment may be the only proven way.

We have heard or shall hear a great deal about individual rights—about conflicts of interest, invasion of privacy, informed consent, least restrictive intervention, rights to treatment, and rights to refuse treatment. This is new in the annals of medicine because prior to the 20th century the sufferer was expected to relinquish personal rights as he submitted himself to care in a child-like patient role. In the past, the physician has assumed the role of parent or guardian, which could and would exercise the patient's rights. As you know, the physician could be trusted in this role because he eschewed all other powers and advantage and had taken an oath to not kill, harm, or break confidence. As a boy, I remember what I am sure was not an isolated event when doctors in my grandfather's generation were asked by the head nurses of general hospital medical wards which of their adult ambulatory patients should be allowed to vote! As a young psychiatrist I remember being asked which chronic patients were competent to vote. Even at the beginning of the 1980s psychiatrists are still being asked to advise the courts about competence to stand trial and competence to manage personal affairs.

The entire medical common law of patient rights, contractual obligation, negligence, liability, and duty of care belongs to the 20th century. Although in many ways these rights developments have reduced the parental or authoritative role of the physician, the goal of rights development has been to establish equity for the patients. Rights of the patient seem to complement the restraint of clinical power of the physician by professional ethics. Rights define immunities and privileges assignable to those at disadvantage. Both the public image of the physician's ethics and the patient's rights appear to have the same teleological basis: establishment in the doctor/patient relationship of transection equity. *The most powerful person is restrained by ethics, the weaker is compensated by rights.*

The application of rights is almost the obverse of the Athenian way. In the time of Pericles, rights were attempts to define standards of equality among the privileged few who were already part of the "democracy." In the 20th century, rights essentially have come to define the furthest limits of suffrage. The limits are now extended to the sick and disabled, and the rights provide privileges and immunities which raise the functional status of the disabled individual to full constitutional or equal protection and access to due process. At the present time we are debating whether full or partial rights will even be extended to children, born or unborn. *These newer rights are no longer standards of equality among equals, but equalizers among unequals.* This suggests a conclusion of the Age of Enlightenment with the universal suffrage abhorred by Aristotle and foreseen by J. S. Mill. Each citizen, whether weak or strong, adult or child, wise or foolish, would be equally secure in the womb and to the tomb. Wherever we find inequity, we presume existence of some form of rights violation, therefore new rights will continue to be created until we run out of classes of people suspect of deprivation. No one person can be entrusted to administer and enforce them. There must be enough courts, lawyers, process servers, police, peer reviewers, and civil servants to handle all of the forms. An attorney or guardian *ad litem* would be needed for every case manager-client transaction. Alternatively, the ethical code could obligate each manager to exercise each right on the behalf of the client. A third alternative would place far less emphasis on client rights and more on a code of professional deportment which assures a high minded exclusive dedication to client's welfare. The first alternative would be the slowest and most cumbersome. Judges would be the ultimate clinical decision-makers. The second would result in a scenario somewhat like the following:

> Mary, this is Joe, your case manager. I have a prescription a doctor wrote for you and I think you should take it. But first, I must tell you all about the dangers and risks involved and also about alternative treatments that might be more effective. You must not take it for the one or more years it will take to have an attorney appointed, to advocate every conceivable opposition in a public trial where the doctor's and my credibility can be challenged and cross-examined so that the court is assured that your rights are not violated. I do not assume, Mary, that your failure to answer me is a silent assent of any kind to the treatment I have proposed.

The third alternative could result in a transaction such as the following:

> Dear Mr. Jones: Your sister and ward, Mary, has been seen by Dr. Smith, a physician in whom I have complete confidence. He has pre-

scribed schizomycin, and after careful review I have concluded that this treatment will provide her the maximum chance of recovery with the least risk of unfavorable side-effects and with least restriction of her freedom. Unless you notify me of any objections you may have to this treatment, I will arrange for her to begin taking the medicine ten days from now. You can be sure that the good effect of the treatment will be carefully followed by me and that I will contact you immediately if it appears that any changes will be necessary.

In regard to your offer to contribute to the Case Manager's Study Retreat, I want to express appreciation, but regret that my colleagues and I are ethically unable to accept any favors or benefit from you or others whom we are obliged to serve without compensation beyond the handsome stipend already provided us by law. Of course, your contribution to a Case managers' Professional Program in another state would be acceptable and very much welcomed. Sincerely yours, (The Honorable) _____ _____, Case Manager

The first two alternatives would be impractical and probably not worth the money and effort required to train case managers. The last alternative would possibly work if the public could shift focus from a rights approach to inequity to a reverent reliance on scholarship and public commitment by managers to ethical deportment. However unpalatable or old-fashioned such an approach might be, it may be the only way[1] to avoid counterproductive if not hopeless case non-management.

Summary and Conclusions

There is no precedent for the natural inequality of an effective physician-patient relationship or case manager-client relationship which is compensated by enforcement of constitutional rights. Outside enforcement displaces the healing or comforting function of the relationship so that there is compliance, not management or care. Implementation and coordination of state services and fund raising for private services are almost insurmountable tasks even for the case manager with consummate political skills, let alone the manager who will have no powers to enforce agency cooperation. Case management ethics based entirely on adherence to client

---

[1]The client advocacy potential of managers totally committed to client welfare would be obvious (if not threatening) to government agencies and private interests in conflict with client rights.

rights would make fulfillment of a powerless job responsibility impossible. Experience of pre-19th-century powerless physicians suggests that a strong public commitment to high ethical deportment and restraint in the exercise of a client's rights might provide a powerless manager a means of enhancing patient cooperation, job viability, and personal survival until it can be shown that deinstitutionalization and community-based care can be sustained with individualized management.

Part IV

TRAINING CASE MANAGERS

Chapter 8

THE EXPERIENCE IN NEW YORK STATE

Michael Ross, Ph.D.
Nancy Riffer, Ph.D.
Tim Switalski

Introduction and Background

Case Management training has evolved in the past several years in New York State in the context of the changing policy environment of the State Office of Mental Health (OMH). It was born out of a need to promote the concepts of what has come to be known as the Community Support Program (CSP). It was developed at a time when the state legislature and the control agencies (Budget and Civil Service) were making initial budgetary and bureaucratic commitments to the spawning of a large, new alternative system of support and care in the community. It was delivered at a time when the Office of Mental Health began moving large sums of money to pay for these new support services to community agencies, county mental health services, and its own facilities. It was evaluated and analyzed at a time when the Office of Mental Health began to turn away the CSP model, and it is being revised at this writing at a time when the Office is struggling to adopt the Balanced Service System (BSS) model in place of CSP. All this in two years time.

Prior to June 1977, OMH did not officially acknowledge the need for case management services and therefore had no organized training program. Today, it spends approximately $4 million on these services. It has 314 persons officially performing them and another 500 or so performing them out of title at one level of professional competence or another. It has spent $250,000 on developing and delivering case management training since 1977 and has budgeted another $250,000 in 1979/80 alone for training another 325 persons. It is truly a growth industry in New York.

The Office of Mental Health, of course, has no monopoly on the concepts, the practice, and, one supposes, the training of case managers. Before 1977, many persons were providing these services to their clients, au-thorized or not, in one agency or another, under one auspice or another, simply because it made good sense to do so. These hearty pioneers may have had some formal training in a local college or university, at a school of social work, or even at an occasional workshop. The conceptual baggage was also not new, having rattled around in one form or another in the social work literature. Indeed, before CSP seized on it as the linchpin of community support, Balanced Services and its intellectual forefathers had made it the rim of its system wheel.

The impact of this evolving policy environment on case management services and training in New York is the single most important factor influencing the shape and content of the training we have today. In the summer of 1977, the policy-makers then in charge of the Office of Mental Health faced the need to impact quickly and profoundly on the way mental health services were being delivered in the state. As in most states, these services were largely dominated by the activities of the state hospitals, or psychiatric centers as they had come to be called. There were (and are) county-based mental health services and numerous free-standing voluntary agencies servicing OMH clients on contract. Of course, some of the psychiatric centers had community-based services of one type or another. Still, more than 80% of the OMH budget was committed to facility- or hospital-based, inpatient services.

All of this was in the face of the very extensive deinstitutionalization of OMH clients in the 1970s which saw a decline in hospital population from 75,000 persons in 1970 to 28,000 in 1977. This rapid and often unplanned evacuation of the state hospitals led to the saturation of some communities with large numbers of uncared for and unsupported former residents of state hospitals, often unable to cope with community living. In this context, CSP, which was then emerging as the new national consensus on how to deliver comprehensive community mental health services, was adopted by OMH leadership and supported by the principal political figures in the state.

Central to the community support system approach was case manage-ment. In New York, a major commitment was made to the widespread employment of case management services as a means of rapidly improving the ability of clients to cope with community life. In effect, a decision was made by OMH with the concurrence of the political leadership and the control agencies to invest rapidly and heavily in a statewide version of the community support program and in particular to rely on case management all over the state to alleviate the more pressing problems felt by clients and communities. Though New York was the recipient in 1977 of the largest award under the new NIMH Community Support Program, its own commitment to CSS turned out to be much more than a demonstration or pilot project.

In view of these interwoven political, planning, and service considerations, it was necessary to develop a training design that closely promoted the goals of the principal policy-makers of the Office of Mental Health. Hence, it was decided that the training design should have four major features. It should:

1. be based on a uniform and consistent job design of how case management services were to be delivered;
2. have a common curriculum describing the functions, duties, roles, activities, and tasks of the job;
3. be skill oriented, utilizing training devices that promote an integration of theory and practice in the work place;
4. be locally deliverable, employing local trainers, known to and respected by the local providers. A minimum of central administration and intervention was to be necessary to deliver the training in numerous sites simultaneously all over the state.

With these goals in mind, the Director of the CSS Manpower Development and Training Project (one of the authors of this chapter) worked closely with the policy-makers and the relevant technical units from the beginning of the design and development process. He joined with the Director of Personnel and others with manpower responsibility in the design of the job description for the new case managers. This involvement at the earliest stage of design was an unusual and happy occurrence in New York. Instead of being presented with a training problem to solve where often the program design had been completed, the training staff was involved in the program design itself. It also had the opportunity to influence the thinking of the program, personnel, and manpower units from the training perspective.

Several fateful decisions were made in this design phase that have greatly influenced case management services in New York State. It was decided that a new civil service title should be established to deliver these services, instead of using existing titles, unchanged or modified. It was also decided that this new title, eventually called *Community Client Service Assistant* (CCSA), was to be established at a paraprofessional grade level. A number of political, clinical, and policy considerations influenced these decisions. From a clinical point of view, it was felt that the principal need of clients living in the community was for a single person to assist them on a day-to-day basis to cope with community living, supplementing their own missing or atrophied life management skills. Such a person was to have a "street wise" sense of life, willing to work with clients face-to-face in the often tedious routine experienced by them. It was felt that a paraprofessional with the proper experience and training would have more than adequate skills for such work and might even have superior job-related attitudes as well. From a political point of view, it was felt that an opportunity for career advancement for the lowest level inpatient, hospital staff (Mental Health Therapy Aide) should be provided for community-based work, in view of the commitment to reduce the size of the hospital component of the state's mental health system and in consideration of the commitment to continuity of employment made to the Civil Service Union. It was also believed that persons with this type of inpatient experience might be especially well suited to perform the functions envisioned for the new Community Client Service Assistant. Finally, budgetary constraints influenced the size of the pay level that could reasonably be contemplated by OMH in view of the large, expanding manpower commitment that was envisioned for the future. The decision to use a new title in the first place was made on the calculation that, while existing titles already described case management services intermixed with numerous, other essential non-case management functions, the case managers that were needed would have to perform *only* case management functions to be certain that clients received the necessary linking, advocacy, monitoring, facilitating, and helping functions needed for their survival in the community.

Two other fateful decisions were made at this point that greatly influenced the shape and content of the training. It was decided that the CCSAs were not to engage in the delivery of organized therapeutic services nor to be responsible on their own for service planning and assessment functions. Numerous factors, clinical and otherwise, conspired to produce this decision. In the end, it was felt that the highest priority need was for staff to supplement the missing life management skills of clients, and not for additional manpower to do therapy and to plan and assess. In fact, it was felt that properly organized *case management programs* could round out existing therapy, planning, and assessment resources with the new additional CCSA items. The literature in the field seemed also to support the notion that the client level, face-to-face linking, advocacy, and monitoring functions envisioned for the CCSAs were not compatible with the therapeutic relationship and would be so time-consuming as to leave little time for service planning and assessment. These functions, it was felt, should be assigned to supervisors of case managers with professional credentials.

Development and Design of the Training

In view of these numerous considerations and in view of the training goals, it was decided that the training should be delivered from a comprehensive training package made up of a manual, a workbook, and support materials. The training was to be delivered by locally hired trainees with education and experience in the delivery of community-based mental health services. These trainers were to be assigned cohorts of trainees ranging in size from six to ten persons, working in case management programs near enough to each other to meet one afternoon a week for (what turned out to be) a sequence of 14 weeks. Each sequence was to be regarded as a training cycle. Groups of cycles were programmed to begin in each region of the state simultaneously as the case managers (CCSAs) were hired. Each cycle was to be equipped with all the instructional materials it would need to function more or less self-sufficiently during the 14 weeks. To prepare the trainers to use these materials, they were brought together themselves in each region for three days of intensive training.

To initiate each training cycle, the case managers from an entire region were also brought together to a two-day orientation conference. During this conference, they were taught their job duties and roles, the structure of the support services being made available to clients in their local community, and the values underlying their work with clients. These sessions worked best when they met during the conference with the trainer who would lead their local training group after the conference.

The training of the case manager is based on helping him to understand the community support system and his role in helping clients function in the community.

The functions of the case manager were described in terms of eight roles: facilitator, linker, supporter, broker, monitor, bridger, catalyst, and advocate. These roles were defined as follows:

facilitator: to make the client's interaction with the system work more easily

linker: to bring clients and services together at the client level including making introductions, communicating, providing information, following up supporter: to show caring to the client and confidence in the client's ability to take more responsibility for his life

broker: to help the client obtain the services he needs, which may include negotiating on his behalf

monitor: to follow up to see that client and services are doing what they have agreed to

bridger: to build bridges where there are gaps—between clients, clients and agencies, or service providers in one agency and those in another

catalyst: to bring problems to the attention of others so that they initiate actions which lead to changes for clients

advocate: to assist the client in defending his rights as a client and as a citizen

These roles describe the different styles in which the case manager was to operate to bring clients and services together in ways which result in the increased empowerment of the client.

In addition, job duties were specified in terms of those with whom the case manager relates—the client, the treatment and discharge staff, the providers of human services, the providers of commercial services, the client's family and friends, and the supervisor. The variety of activities that the case manager would engage in to help the client manage his life and utilize services in the community was discussed.

The description of the community support system and of the job duties and roles was accompanied by orientation to the values which underlie case management for the chronically mentally disabled. These were:

1. Clients should receive the *appropriate level of care*.
2. Increasingly, *community-based services* should be available to clients.
3. Clients should receive aid in learning the skills they need to fulfill their highest potential through rehabilitation.
4. The value of *normalization* means that clients should be treated as closely as possible to the way others who are "normal" are treated, e.g., they should receive services in normal settings, not psychiatric settings.
5. Services should be provided to clients in ways which *empower the client*—which enable him to see himself as active in his environment and as making a difference in his own life.
6. Clients should be encouraged to be *self-reliant and responsible*.

The goal in teaching these values is to show how to build a community support system which is responsive to the needs of individual clients and which enables each one to find a way in which he can live in the community. The challenge for the CCSA is to find a balance between the provision of services which are so inclusive that they envelop the clients and services which put clients on their own in the community with too few resources.

Following the conference, case managers met in their half day per week sessions for 14 weeks. These sessions had two major foci: (1) the learning of theory and skills which were seen as basic to the case management function and (2) the integration of theory and practice through discussions based on a structured field experience. Theory and skill topics included discharge planning, goal setting, and problem solving with clients; basic values in rehabilitation; the local providers in the community support system; skills as a supporter/facilitator; adult learning theory; complying with agency processes; psychopharmacological treatments; recognizing gaps and dysfunctions in the client's support system; accessing information on available human services; advocacy; client behavior in the community; conflict resolution; preventing burnout of case managers; and a 6-week unit on basic helping skills. Two to three hours of each seminar session were spent covering these topics through lectures, discussions, forums, role-playing, agency visits, case analyses, etc. The training manual, *Case Management Services in Community Support Systems,* contained all the basic information for these sessions.

Simultaneously, case managers were asked to focus on their work with a selected client. They were guided in this by the *Constructive Action Workbook.* This workbook is an adaptation of the basic process used by the College for Human Services in New York City to educate its human services graduates. In the constructive action designed for this training, the case manager was to focus on the process of delivering a major piece of service to a particular client he and his supervisor selected and to reflect on and articulate this process in written assignments and seminar discussions.

The work with the client over the 14 weeks falls into three phases: planning, implementation, and assessment. To *plan* for work with the client each case manager is directed to know (1) his own job description, (2) the mandate of his agency, (3) the client with whom he reaches an agreement to work, (4) the goals the client is willing to work toward, (5) the goals the work supervisor recommends in working with this client, and (6) the learning he needs to do to be able to aid this client effectively. To *implement* the plan of action arrived at by the case manager, the client, the work supervisor, and the trainer together, the case manager aggregates the necessary resources from within and outside his agency, pursues his learning goals, supports the client in the community, and revises the goals as necessary. The *assessment* phase focuses on how successfully the case manager has met the service and learning goals set in the plan of action and in later modifications.

The constructive action involves working with the client, preparing written descriptions and analyses of what happened with the client each week, and discussing these experiences during training sessions. Further, the trainer observes the case manager in the field at least once and keeps in touch with the work supervisor about the case manager's progress.

The training group of six to ten case managers became the setting within which skills were practiced and problems discussed. The case managers were encouraged to use their co-workers and their trainer as resources for improving the service they were providiang. Teamwork and peer support were considered to be the keys to the success of the case managers.

The trainers hired in each region were familiar with the resources, politics, and service systems in their locality. They were recommended by the regional office and by local service providers. The three-day trainer conference held in each region to orient the trainers to the curriculum also provided an opportunity for trainers, work supervisors, and service agency directors to reach agreement on the local implementation of training. The general curriculum in the manual was used to shape the training in line with statewide objectives. Speakers, case histories, and training group discussions were used to adapt the curriculum to local circumstances.

Focus on the Trainer

The role of the trainer in the case management program has proven to be challenging and frustrating. Case management functions were as new to the trainees as they were to the agencies within which they were working. It was important that the trainers be able to communicate effectively to both groups to insure that the training reflected the needs of the case managers and their agency employers. To accomplish this, trainers were selected who had a working knowledge of the human service system in their community and who felt comfortable embracing the case management concept.

The material to be used throughout the program was distributed to the trainers prior to their own training so that they could familiarize themselves with the curriculum. The trainers in each region met with each other and with the curriculum developers to explore the values and philosophy underlying case management and to discuss methods and techniques to be used in conducting the training. This "trainer training" session was crucial in helping the trainers to "own" the material and to incorporate their knowledge, skills, and experience into the curriculum design.

The inclusion of agency directors and case management work supervisors in the trainer conference added another dimension to their perspective. Issues relating to the local implementation of training were negotiated at this time, and the role of the work supervisor in the training program was defined. In the original design this role was to be left to the local trainers and agencies to work out.

Group dynamics began to develop in the introductory conference when trainers began functioning as leaders whose behavior and attitudes would then be emulated by the trainees. It became increasingly important for trainers to demonstrate commitment to the case management concept, the training program, and its usefulness to the trainees to keep up morale in the face of the many problems new service and training programs usually face. Trainers had also to demonstrate, early on in the program, that they already had in abundance the skills and knowledge that were the subject of the training so as to establish an appropriate model for their trainees.

As the training progressed through the 14-week program, learning was facilitated in a group interaction process. Case managers were encouraged to review assigned material prior to each session and to participate in discussions which were relevant to their field experience. The use of case presentations, group exercises, and role plays were also useful methods of promoting this process. The trainer would often act as a catalyst in these situations by stimulating the interaction while allowing the participants to explore fully the issues involved. Trainers would often be confronted with individual resistance to this process and had to be prepared to deal with it directly, either within the group or individually.

The Constructive Action offered several opportunities for group interaction around common issues. The phases of planning, implementing, and assessing for a selected client would often lead to discussions of the eight roles of the case manager and would focus discussion on the notion of empowerment. On an individual level this methodology was useful in assessing progress in integrating theory with practice. It also provided a focal point for more intensive discussion between case managers, trainers, and work supervisors.

A critical issue throughout the training was the extent of the flexibility the trainer could exercise in delivering the curriculum. Case managers had different levels of skill and ability as well as a variety of backgrounds. It was difficult to deliver the same curriculum to trainees having different learning needs without making adaptations in the material.

The material to be covered in the curriculum was extensive, making it difficult to devote equal coverage to all topic areas. Trainers were encouraged to make their own judgments as to which areas should receive the most emphasis throughout the training. These judgments were to be based on input received from work supervisors and case managers.

The use of guest speakers who described the functions of community service agencies or made presentations on topics in which they had expertise was found to be informative to case managers and their work supervisors. This proved especially valuable when speakers were familiar with direct services. An option which also proved successful called for case managers to make on-site visits to various agencies and then to discuss their observations in the group during the following session. This option also allowed the visited agencies to learn about the new case management community resource available to them for their clients.

In summary, the role of the case management trainer involved the responsibility for implementing the curriculum in a manner which made the sessions enjoyable, relevant, and beneficial to the case managers in their ongoing practice.

Conclusions

Review of this first round of training for case managers has led to several conclusions:

1. Training to work with individual clients (helping skills, crisis intervention, the relationship of the case manager and the client) and training to work with the system (orientation to special programs for the chronically disabled, information on state and federal programs, advocacy skills, and formal advocacy resources) are the central content areas for case managers.
2. A process for relating theory and practice through field experience is necessary in this kind of training program.
3. In training for participation in a new system, trainees may look to training staff to solve problems that are implementation questions outside their jurisdiction. Trainers are not responsible for solving program issues, yet they have to base training on the realities of the

local situation, not on statements of how things are supposed to operate.

4. Training should be flexible enough to meet the needs of case managers from a wide variety of backgrounds.

5. Trainers need clear direction on what parts of the training must be covered and what choices they have for adapting or substituting materials.

6. The group process in the training groups is central to learning. Sufficient time must be allowed for discussion of experiences and problem solving during weekly training sessions.

7. Assessment of prior learning of case managers is essential to facilitate the adaptation of training to individual skill levels and local needs.

Chapter 9

TRAINING CASE MANAGERS FOR THE DEVELOPMENTAL DISABILITIES SYSTEM

Richard F. Antonak, Ed.D.

The recent Developmental Disabilities Amendments (P.L. 95-602 of 1979) establishes as a top priority the coordination of the complex array of human service agencies, providers, programs, and facilities—public, private, and proprietary—generic and specific—in the interests of the developmentally disabled citizen. In Wolf Wolfensberger's PASS model, this is referred to as *model coherency*; that is, insuring that the developmentally disabled individual receives the right services in a timely and normalized manner by the right provider in the most appropriate setting to maximize the individual's developmental potential. This concept, and its associated system, has many names; the one which is most common and the one used in this book is *case management.*

My purpose in this chapter is not to analyze or define the case management system—I will leave that to my distinguished colleagues represented in this book. Rather, I want to share with you some thoughts about and recommendations for training case managers for the developmental disabilities service delivery system. As a framework for this discussion, let me attempt to analyze the basis for this professional manpower demand.

Manpower Demand

The passage in 1970 of the Developmental Disabilities Services and Facilities Construction Act (P.L. 91-517), the subsequent Developmental Disabilities Assistance and Bill of Rights Act of 1975 (P.L. 94-103), and the Developmental Disabilities Amendments of 1979 (P.L. 95-602) provided the impetus for change in the delivery of human services to the significantly handicapped, influencing both the population to be served and the nature of the services to be delivered. With regard to the population, it was recognized that the formerly independent groups of disabled individuals (i.e., the mentally retarded, epileptic, cerebral palsied, and autistic) were not functionally independent. The synthesis of these groups was based on the awareness that these conditions have a common temporal and neurological origin, constitute a substantial handicap to the individual, and require similar, though changing, services on a lifelong basis.

The second area of significant change concerned the organization and administration of human service programs. Prior to the Developmental Disabilities (DD) concept, each of the handicapping conditions had engendered interest, advocacy, and lobby groups which competed for scarce resources, but which eventually created or supported service programs and facilities with common objectives (e.g., education, training, occupational competence, medical intervention), common procedures (e.g., applied behavior analysis, task analysis), and common special service providers (e.g., occupational, physical, speech and recreation therapists, educators, counselors). This led to the overlap and duplication of service facilities and programs, restrictive eligibility requirements, and the fractionation of the human service delivery system. The DD concept was seen as a means to overcome these programmatic and administrative tangles, and the tool was the concept of a service delivery system.

New Hampshire statute (RSA 171-A, June 4, 1975) defines a service delivery system as:

> a comprehensive array of services for the diagnosis, evaluation, habilitation, and rehabilitation of developmentally disabled persons, including but not limited to developmental centers, work activity programs, community residences, family care, foster care, day care, and residential care and treatment. . .

While this concept was innovative and clearly necessary to support the DD population synthesis, the development of a comprehensive service delivery system has been slow and tentative. One reason is the necessity to bring together those agencies and advocacy groups which had heretofore competed for resources. The Developmental Disabilities umbrella engendered competition for funds, staff, and support, and the result was strained communication between agencies and disciplines, inadequate organization, and services which were non-responsive to client's needs.

Perhaps a more telling reason for the delay in generating a comprehensive service delivery system has been the acute lack of adequately trained manpower. The current emphasis on deinstitutionalization and the creation of alternative community services has created two manpower needs nationally. One need is at the paraprofessional level; that is, for supervised personnel to provide direct services to developmentally disabled citizens as they progress through the service delivery system. The state of Maine has addressed this DD manpower need with its Community Client Services Assistant (or CCSA) model—a paraprofessional trained at the associate degree level through a series of 12 weekly training sessions of 4 to 5 hours each. The New York State program (presented by my colleagues) is directed to a similar need in the mental health service delivery system.

The second manpower need, at the unit management level, requires professionals who are trained to assume administrative, supervisory, and management roles in an array of settings and community-based facilities for developmentally disabled persons. Moreover, this manpower need entails both preservice preparation of professionals to enter the system and also retraining of professionals who currently find themselves in the role of case manager. It is toward this unit level case management manpower need in Developmental Disabilities that the University of New Hampshire is directing its attention.

Program Description

Proposal Development

A group of interested faculty members from the Department of Education of the College of Liberal Arts and from the Departments of Communication Disorders and Occupational Therapy of the School of Health Studies collaborated to prepare a proposal for a Master's Degree program in Developmental Disabilities. This proposal represented the examination of professional preparation programs offered elsewhere in the nation, careful analysis of federal and state legislation, a survey of New England regional and New Hampshire manpower needs, and the input of a statewide and regional advisory committee consisting of representatives of each state's disability advocacy groups (UCPA, EFA, NARC, NSAC), the State Department of Education, the State Department of Mental Health and Developmental Services, the Region I HEW Office, the New England region UAFs, and administrators of direct service agencies serving the developmentally disabled from across the state.

The case management concept on which this training program was based presumed a special series of considerations which are not common in case management models for social services, mental health, or rehabilitation. In particular, the needs of the developmentally disabled are lifelong, substantial, and most often multiple. The case management functions must therefore begin as early as possible with aggressive casefinding, integrate a diversity of human services in a sequential manner with shifting emphasis over time, and continue indefinitely. Case closure will rarely occur in a DD case management system. Continuity of service, concern, and attention, from service phase to service phase, throughout the life of the developmentally disabled individual is essential. This responsibility was determined to be most appropriately assigned to a Master's level professional called a case manager.

Professional Skills

The training program was designed to accept Bachelor's-level professionals from a variety of human service disciplines—education; occupational, physical, speech, recreation therapy; nursing; health administration; social service; psychology—and provide them with the skills, knowledge, and attitudes to relate to their peers in other human service disciplines in constructive, client-centered manners. While it is recognized that the human service delivery system will evolve over time, generic competencies can be identified and grouped into three broad categories:

Administrative-Management Skills and Knowledge

- knowledge of systems theory
- system assessment and evaluation skills
- maintaining a resource directory for I & R
- recordkeeping and reporting
- sequencing and scheduling
- management information systems knowledge
- resource mobilization skills
- quality assurance/accountability knowledge
- fiscal management skills - resource procurement
- knowledge of current regulations, eligibility requirements, policy
- service broker skills
- knowledge of the political process - lobbying
- communitization skills - resource development
- skills to promote interagency coordination

Human Relations Skills and Knowledge

- methods of attitude change
- social welfare process and theory - policy analysis
- interpersonal skills - conferences, interviews, teaming
- communication theory and process knowledge
- group theory/process/dynamics
- observation skills
- consulting skills
- problem-solving skills

Clinical Skills

- knowledge of causes, characteristics, and treatments for developmental disabilities
- knowledge of human development, learning theory
- knowledge of human service delivery system concepts
- knowledge of an array of human service disciplines
- aggressive outreach - case finding skills
- service needs assessment, problem definition
- profiling strengths and weaknesses
- service planning - ISP writing - goal setting
- referral for detailed evaluation and diagnosis
- linking clients to services/arranging/connecting/bridging
- knowledge of client rights and entitlements
- skills in advocacy
- skills in tracking, follow-along, overseeing
- crisis intervention skills

Program Organization

In planning the training program, an attempt was made to provide sufficient flexibility for graduate students to design a course of study which ensures the development of the necessary skills and competencies but which also incorporates previous professional training and practical experience. Accordingly, the program is organized into three phases. The first phase consists of a set of core courses on (a) human learning and development; (b) the history, characteristics, and treatment of the developmentally disabled; (c) administration of human service delivery systems; and (d) the concepts of systems theory and service delivery systems. A series of elective courses are available from among a wide range of courses offered by graduate programs in education, business administration, psychology, sociology, public administration, recreation, vocational rehabilitation, and others.

The second phase entails a series of biweekly seminars in which specific topics are addressed relating to the development, administration, evaluation, and modification of human service delivery systems. These topics typically include deinstitutionalization, the legislative process, PASS, communitization, advocacy, etc. To facilitate the student's understanding of the various programs and the professional disciplines he or she will be encountering, a second seminar series is offered which provides an intensive survey of the terminology, theory, and clinical practice of a diversity of human service providers. Guest lecturers from state and regional service facilities and programs provide a base from which the seminar coordinator focuses the students' discussion on the sharing, communication, and interdependence required for interdisciplinary program planning for developmentally disabled individuals.

The final phase of the program entails a two-part field practicum. The first half of the practicum consists of a series of experiences in a diversity of programs and facilities which provide services for the developmentally disabled. In addition, the student observes, interacts with, and assists professionals engaged in the delivery of the full array of human services. The second half of the practicum permits an encompassing experience with a particular program for case management experience. Supervised placements are located in which the student gradually increases his or her participation until he or she is approximating the duties of a full-time professional. Supervision is provided by university faculty and field supervisors, and the student is required to meet a set of minimum competencies in the areas previously listed. To complete the degree, the student is required to complete successfully a comprehensive examination designed in accordance with the students graduate program experiences.

Conclusion

Although the case management training program presented is designed to address a significant manpower need in developmental disabilities, there remains a number of issues which require constant attention and clarification as the system evolves. The skills which these professionals may need to perform the case management functions adequately are certainly more than those which the program can include as terminal objectives. The keys to the success of the program are the quality, scope, and depth of the coursework and the content of the seminars and practicum experiences. The necessity to establish priorities on certain skills and competencies and the trade-offs which are required in terms of availability of practica sites, time constraints, student selection criteria, and resource allocation will determine how effective the graduate will be in serving the state's developmentally disabled citizens. The program is committed to change in response to feedback solicited from a variety of sources and will attempt to feedforward to prepare best those professionals needed to function as case managers in the evolving developmentally disabilities service delivery system.

Part V

REHABILITATION

Chapter 10

A PROCESS WITHIN A SYSTEM

Linda Lyman

Who are you? What motivated you to read this book? What is your philosophy – your purpose? What's important to you? Is your identity – a position – a title – a role? What happens to your identity when your position, title, or role is threatened? How do you handle change? Where do your supports come from? How do your learn? How do you grow and develop? How do you help others to learn who they are and how do you support their growth? Can you accept your own limitations and can you help others to accept theirs without anger or guilt? Are you a protector, rescuer, enabler, facilitator? Can you respond to where others are in their own development? Can you expect more of yourself without pressure and see crisis and demanding unmet needs as an opportunity for growth—your growth? Are you in touch with your own power? Can you allow others the power of efficacy? Does your satisfaction come from seeing others take charge of their own lives or are you a little threatened that they no longer need you? Where do your strength and energy come from? Are you adventuresome? Can you take risks? Can you dare to care—when others are too comfortable to change? Are you flexible? What happens to you when your autonomy is threatened? Do not put value judgments on your answers to these questions.

Think of yourself as an intricate organization, and take some time to reflect on how your systems operate. Take the normal, healthy emotion anger as an example. When you feel anger inside, what happens to your affect, behavior, thinking process, other emotions? Do you express your anger or deny it? Do you withdraw? How do you handle resentment? Do you become aggressive? Are you rational, realistic? How does your anger affect others?

How does your agency, center, department, team, or board organizational system operate? Who has the real power? Who has the believability? How is anger dealt with? Openly and honestly or is it not allowed to surface? Where are the supports? What are the meanings of the games that are played? How is trust established? How do you get approval? How is accountability handled? Who delegates responsibility? How does your agency handle change? Is burnout an issue? How is it handled? How much time do you spend in meetings talking about what you ought to be doing? How do you measure outcome? Is that the end result of your efforts? What is the creditability of your center in your community or catchment area?

How does your center fit into the larger health care system within your state? How does your center relate to the state system? What creditability role does your center play in the state system? How is your center recognized or rewarded for its creditability? Who determines your center's autonomy? Reflect, if you will, on how you directly influence your center's organizational system, the creditability of health care in your community, and the larger, though distant, mental health state system!

Or is it, do you think, the other way around—that the state system influences you? Or are you, your center, your board, your community, the state system involved equally in a cooperative, autonomous mental health movement?

I hope your answers to these questions will help you in the process of defining and implementing case management for you, your center, your community, *and* most particularly your clients. *Case management is a process within a system.* I believe that if general systems theory is better understood, the chances for survival and success of any changes, within a given system, are much greater.

In a treatment setting, a mental health center, or the community at large, a wide range of treatment methods should be available to be used for the clients' benefit in an integrated way, for example, job counselors, social club or group leaders, house managers, medical personnel, family therapist, and case manager. I suggest that there should be a complex set of continuous, dynamic relationships between everyone connected to the client if the treatment plan is going to attempt to meet all of the clients' needs.

Many a well thought out client care plan has failed because the various professionals were unable to work together toward a common goal. The psychiatric patient preparing to re-enter the mainstream of responsible community living has problems in so many different areas that it is impossible for one professional worker to become an expert in everything. Interdisciplinary cooperation is necessary.

Enthusiasm for and control of the case management process must extend from the very top of the administration hierarchy to every member of the treatment team. It is essential to realize that we all have built-in resistance to change. There will always be some reluctance to try out new ideas and procedures. Perhaps the most difficult resistance to deal with is apparent cooperation which covers an underlying hostility and lack of understanding. There is nothing more destructive to the ultimate establishment of a new approach than the hidden resistance of a self-fulfilling and actually self-defeating prophecy: the unexpressed and therefore especially potent attitude that case management won't work in our community, of if it is possible, it's not worth the effort, leads to unobstructive undermining of the plans. The moods, fears, anxieties, conflicts, depressions of each person in the system will affect the others if these emotional forces are strong enough. Within the milieu setting, staff mental health has a direct correlation to patient mental health.

The Thresholds Program/Process

I have a poster hanging on my office which pictures a man rowing a boat. The caption reads: "If there is not wind . . . Row!" This is our aim at Thresholds: To help our members overcome the hopelessness often associated with mental illness, to learn that almost anything can be accomplished if the will to do it exists. The key to Thresholds' philosophy is the rebuilding of self-motivation and self-confidence.

Thresholds is a rehabilitation center for former psychiatric patients in Chicago. We are celebrating our 20th anniversary this year. Our clients are called members, their ages range from 16-50. There are about 225 members in the program at any one time. Members are referred by social service agencies, private therapists, state and private psychiatric hospitals, mental health clinics, the Division of Vocational Rehabilitation, the Board of Education, family, or self-referral.

Our original center is located on Chicago's north side, across the street from Lincoln Park overlooking Lake Michigan. This warm, Adler-designed mansion is a non-institutional setting providing the environment ideally suited to promote transition from mental illness to mental health.

Our membership falls into three groupings: The young adults, 16-21 years old; the mothers' project with their children ranging in age from 1 month to 6 years; and our general membership. All members participate to some extent in our multi-faceted program designed to bring the emotionally disturbed back into the mainstream of community living through the achievement of our five major goals: vocational rehabilitation, social rehabilitation, academic preparation, independent living, prevention of rehospitalization. All members are part of the milieu—the pulse of our program.

One-fourth of our day membership is involved in the academic program five mornings a week. Each member has an individualized curriculum designed to meet his needs after initial diagnostic testing. In the same classroom, one member may be working on specific courses to meet credit requirements for graduation from his hometown high school; another member may be preparing to take the GED examination to acquire a high school diploma; still other members, prospective college students, may be boning up for entrance exams. Some members with learning disabilities or perceptual problems or the few who are illiterate are upgrading their basic math and reading skills. Every member is given a reading examination to determine his level of concentration and comprehension. It's important that members can read job application forms and understand basic survival communication. Our school is fully accredited by the Illinois State Board of Education as an alternative school. The school was developed because there were no community resources available for the emotionally disturbed older adolescent or young adult.

Some members need a reason to get up everyday; others need to work to support themselves and to feel a sense of worth. Few psychiatric patients have the confidence to return to their old job or to find a new job directly following a hospitalization. The Thresholds vocational work crew program prepares members for work by teaching good work habits, how to handle responsibility and pressure on the job, and how to establish vocational goals. The relationship between the crew supervisor and members is a strong catalyst for behavioral change, the building of trust and self-confidence. Our work crew responsibilities are vital and necessary for the smooth agency functioning. The reception crew handles a complex telephone system and ongoing fund raising projects. The catering crew plans, shops, prepares, serves, and cleans up after a daily noon meal for members and staff. The maintenance and housekeeping crew keep the building clean and orderly.

The next vocational step is a transitional job placement in the community. The member has demonstrated in the crew that he can handle pressure, responsibility, and a work relationship. A few members begin in a volunteer placement where the expectation is not as high as when one is paid a salary. Other members, more confident but still needing support and supervision, work with a Thresholds staff member on a group placement. Those members ready to work without close supervision will be placed on a 20- or 40-hour-a-week job placement. After a member has been on a placement, three to seven weeks, he is assisted in getting his own job or getting into a special training program, i.e., auto training or secretarial skills. While members are working on a transitional job, they attend weekly evening group meetings to discuss job related problems and issues. Thresholds staff created the transitional job placement program because the mental health stigma prevented members from finding their own jobs. An Employers Council was formed to maintain positive relationships with employers.

Three afternoons and two evenings a week members attend social groups. Our members come to Thresholds feeling isolated, lonely, unable to take risks for fear of rejection. Learning to listen to others, expressing oneself, and sharing feelings with others who care are necessary for meaningful relationships. Our social program falls into three groupings:

—*problem solving:* going through the process of learning to solve problems, make decisions, establish goals, and look for alternatives;
—*activity groups:* athletics, body dynamics, cooking classes, making video films, growing things in the greenhouse;
—*interest groups:* separate sexuality and awareness groups for men and women and other groups that focus on independent living skills.

Generally when members are referred to Thresholds, they are not living independently. Few members have learned the necessary skills to live comfortably in the community. The Thresholds residence program teaches members how to cope with community living at various levels of sophistication. Three group homes are maintained by members who do the food shopping and prepare the meals. Two of the homes have live-in staff. As a more independent step we provide ten furnished apartments in one building, housing 18 members, with no live-in staff. Ten CHA single apartments and other Thresholds apartments in the area provide the last step toward independent living. Thresholds also maintains two hotel rooms a block away from the agency for crisis intervention.

Thresholds staff created the residential program because there were no community resources available to meet the needs of the recovering psychiatric patient. Nursing homes, shelter care homes, and the individual member's parents' house identified the member as being sick and incompetent and did not teach the member the necessary skills to move on toward independence. The prevention of rehospitalization is an important goal for all of us to strive for. It is costly both in dollars and self-esteem for a member to return to the hospital. Case managers make sure members learn to cope in the community and how to develop a supportive social network.

Three psychiatric consultants provide weekly medication management. Our nurse and one of the psychiatrists lead a weekly medication group for members who need to understand better how their own medication affects their biological and emotional system. When one family member is experiencing pain and stress, every family member, even the pets, experiences stress. Thresholds offers an orientation group for parents and spouses, a 10-week supportive group, a parents alumni group, and family therapy for individual families.

No more than 20% of our members are seen on an intensive psychotherapy basis. The major emphasis is on case management. The role of the case manager is to navigate the member through the program helping him to make the most of his rehabilitation opportunities. Meshing all the educational, social, vocational, and residential opportunities within Thresholds, and within the community, into a coherent rehabilitation plan that works for the member is no easy task.

In those early pioneering days of Thresholds, there were no community resources for the recovering psychiatric patient. Thresholds staff had to become creative and innovative to meet the needs of patients being discharged at an alarming rate into the greater Chicagoland area. Everyone heard the Department of Mental Health was discharging 7,000 patients from their hospital system, but the community did not know how to be prepared.

Thresholds is divided into three teams; each team acts like a mini-agency within the larger system and consists of seven case managers, students, and volunteers. The case managers have an average of 10 to 15 active members on their case load. The number of inactive members no longer requiring active service varies greatly among staff. Each team is responsible for meeting the needs of its members; therefore, each team basically has its own residence and apartments, work crew, transitional job placement, social groups, and autonomy. Case managers carry additional responsibilities for the team and agency. All staff are on call seven days a weeks, 24 hours a day. The team leader hires, trains, and supervises all team staff and assumes some major agency administration duties.

I'd like to give you a sketch of the Young Adult team at Thresholds so that you may get a proper perspective.

Diane, working on her Master's degree in Vocational Rehabilitation, has a case load of 17 members, sees the families of most of her members, teaches in the school three mornings a week, and co-leads the Young Adult groups. She is also Chairperson of our Inservice Training Committee which provides weekly training programs for staff.

Cheryl has a Master's degree in Special Education and is working toward a doctorate. As the director of our school, she supervises the other teachers and curriculum consultant as well as coordinating the training for professionals that come to Thresholds to learn our philosophy. Much of her time is spent responding to the educational needs of team members.

Sally is working on her doctorate in Vocational Rehabilitation, supervises our agency group placement, finds transitional job placements for members in the community, and also helps members find their own jobs. In addition she leads the two employment groups for our team and is currently involved in vocational research.

Bruce, a family therapist and ACSW, manages our group house and supervises four live-in staff. He also is co-leader for Young Adult problem-solving groups.

Debby is co-supervisor for the Catering Crew which is comprised of 27 members in two shifts; coordinates the Sustaining Case program, a maintenance group for inactive members who meet three afternoons and one evening a week in a local Presbyterian church; and supervises the students and volunteers that work in Sustaining Care.

Ginni, who has a Master's degree in Vocational Rehabilitation Counseling, is the other co-supervisor for the Catering Crew with responsibility for dealing with the government about commodity food and the Board of Education milk program. In addition to this, she works with the team evening members in a problem-solving group.

Each week the group of case managers sits down together to evaluate members' progress in school, crew, groups, residence, on the job, in the milieu, or with his/her family. Each case manager gets a complete progress report on each member. It is the responsibility of each member and his case manager to work out a realistic rehabilitation plan. Periodically the goals of that plan are reevaluated. Every member must read and sign every monthly progress note and group, crew, school, and resident evaluation form before it goes into his file. If a member is in crisis, the whole team is aware and supportive. All staff members are knowledgeable about that member and his rehab plan and have discussed with the case manager how they will respond to the member in crisis. The case manager also receives a lot of support from co-teammates. That's a comforting feeling.

Case managers are responsible for coordinating all the workers that a member has contact with but in no way feel power and control over them. There is no need to compete—rather to coordinate and complement. A case manager must make a conscious and deliberate effort to develop trusting relationships with other people involved in a member's life. It's important to keep open the channels of communication between workers to eliminate a member's attempt at manipulation. Burnout is not that much of an issue when you can share concern and responsibilities with other workers and agencies you can trust.

We no longer "close cases" at Thresholds. Members no longer needing the day or evening program are put into two categories: medication only and inactive. The case managers work out their own follow-up arrangements with each member on a limited basis—more extensive with some than others. Many members become fully integrated in the community with supportive social systems and resent being contacted so often. If a case manager has made a positive separation at the time a member leaves the program, he will keep in contact and let the case manager know if he is in difficulty and wants help later on. Then there are those few whom you know are depressed or manic and who refuse any assistance from anyone. Those are the times when it becomes clear that the member has the power and control. We can raise expectations, set limits, be supportive and caring, but we cannot control another person's life or behavior.

I will leave these thoughts of Elizabeth Kubler-Ross with you in closing: "To love means not to impose your own powers on your fellowman, but offer him your help. And if he refuses it, to be proud that he can do it on his own strength."

Part VI

CASE STUDIES

INTRODUCTION

This section presents several case studies involving case management in each of the areas of Developmental Disabilities, Community Mental Health, and Welfare. All of these are based on actual case histories, but any information that could reveal the identity of the client has been purposefully disguised and changed to protect his/her right to confidentiality. The cases are to illustrate to the reader the problems and needs of the client system which the establishment of case management is designed to address. These hopefully will serve as a work/study section for trainees as well as a resource guide or reference for those getting their "feet wet" in the case management field. Since these cases involve people from ages 12-80 and cover many different problems, it is my feeling they will be of great help to people to peak their interest in additional and innovative ways to deal with similar situations.

Chapter 11

DEVELOPMENTAL DISABILITIES PROGRAMS

Sandra Pelletier, M.Ed.

CLIENT MANAGEMENT CASE STUDY #1
SAM – AN 18-YEAR-OLD MALE

Reason for Referral: Deinstitutionalization from the state school (after 5 years of residency)

Current Level of Functioning

At the time of his last developmental assessment, Sam was found to be functioning at the developmental levels of 3-4 years in feeding skills, 4 years in dressing skills, and 1-2 years and 6-12 months in receptive and expressive language development. His adaptive behavior functioning was assessed with the AAMD adaptive behavior scale. It was reported that he has achieved relative independence in most areas of self-help. Sam's language development is severely impaired; he does not have any expressive language and indicates most of his needs through gestures and yelling.

Socially, Sam is functioning at approximately the 1-½-year-old level. He is usually compliant to verbal request, but nevertheless he does not initiate or engage in any interactions with others or attempt to perform any tasks independently. With unstructured free time he will engage in repetitive behaviors such as hand flicking and rocking. Occasionally, he will engage in self-injurious behaviors defined as picking at his skin, often of an intensity and duration to cause it to bleed, but he is not aggressive towards others.

Report on Community Placement Status

The state school's interdisciplinary team recommended in 1977 that Sam was a candidate for community placement in a foster home with appropriate educational programming. Attempts had been made to locate a foster home for him by the state school, but they were unsuccessful. In January 1979 this individual was placed on the Client Management Project caseload in order to find a proper community placement. Attempts were made for two months to locate a suitable foster home for him, but this also proved futile.

The Client Management Project had previously arranged for management of a highly supervised living alternative for five mentally retarded individuals in need of a residential setting. Sam was discussed as a possible candidate for this residence. The management of the house is provided by four professional staff on a 3-day rotating basis. Due to Sam's current level of functioning and areas of need, it was felt that placement within this residence was the least restrictive alternative. Sam's father and the state school's interdisciplinary team were in agreement with this residential setting.

The client manager made the proper arrangements needed to guarantee that all the required services for Sam were available in the community or could be made available.

Problems in Obtaining Necessary Services

Guardianship

According to N.H. State Law, RSA 171:A, when a person reaches 18 his/her parents are no longer legal guardians. If Sam's father wished to remain legal guardian, it became necessary for him to initiate guardianship proceedings. Until July 1, 1979 it was required for state school residents to have a legal guardian before community placement could take place. This regulation could in some cases hinder community placement until a guardian could be found or proceedings be completed. The guardianship process at times has taken as long as three months.

In Sam's case, he was placed in the community on extended vacation status until his father completed the proceedings at which time his status was changed to community placement.

Educational Programming

The region has an appropriate program available for adolescents who are severely impaired. However, this program and the other services for the developmentally disabled in this region need to expand in order to accept individuals returning from the state institution. In this region the expansion of existing services alone has not been able to meet the needs; deinstitutionalization has necessitated the creation of new services. It is anticipated that the community will have to develop a continuum of housing alternatives, day programming, and other services in the near future for developmentally disabled individuals.

Companionship Project/Citizen Advocates

Sam's family does not currently reside in this state. Like many other individuals whose families have minimal involvement, the client manager enlists individuals to function in the capacity of a companion. These companions assist the individual who is mentally retarded to become socially integrated into the community. Although the developmentally disabled is now physically located in the community, integration and acceptance are not guaranteed. It is hoped that with the assistance from "normal" peers, community acceptance will be facilitated.

Housing

In order to facilitate successful community placement, in as many cases as possible, a client is brought to the community for short periods (three or four days at a time) for transitional placement. The purpose is not to sever completely the ties from the state school in which many individuals have resided for years. The transitional period also assists community staff in determining if the placement is an appropriate one.

The problem with the transitional procedure is that during this time the client is receiving none of his/her financial benefits (SSI, Welfare, APTD), thus any costs incurred, such as the expense of maintaining the house, staff, etc., are absorbed by the client management project. The client is unable to contribute to his financial welfare until he is placed on community placement status. The cost for transitional placement can range from $15-$30 per day depending on the living alternative.

The needs of Sam had required Client Management to hire additional staff to work directly with him at the house. This became necessary for an interim period of time, to allow him to become accustomed and adjusted to his new situation. He demonstrated behaviors which interfered with programming for the other habitants of this house, thus it became imperative to employ another person to assist. It is hoped that in the near future, the regional system will be able to have in its employ a specialist who will be able to provide intervention. This service would be provided specifically for individuals who have returned from the institution or are currently in the community, who demonstrate management problems which could ultimately lead to an *unsuccessful* community placement and reinstitutionalization.

Financial Assistance

Most individuals returning from the state school are eligible for both Social Security Income and Welfare Aid to the Permanently and Totally Disabled (APTD) benefits. Obtaining these benefits has been one of the major barriers in development caseload. The bureaucratic paperwork, eligibility criteria, and, most of all, the confusion of Welfare and Social Security Offices on how to deal with individuals who are being deinstitutionalized have made this process of obtaining these funds almost an impossibility. Eventually the individual receives his benefits, but often times not until 3-6 months from date of application. All benefits are retroactive; however, in the interim of many months, most client management funds are tied up in maintaining the individual until his funds are released. This process creates a tremendous cash flow problem for the client management system.

CLIENT MANAGEMENT CASE STUDY #2
SALLY – A 23-YEAR-OLD FEMALE

Reason for Referral: This individual was referred by the Office of Mental Retardation. Individual is currently receiving no services and has only received minimal services in the past 23 years. Situation is considered CRISIS. A complete service plan is needed for this individual.
Diagnosis: Moderate mental retardation, no genetic mechanism present; hydrocephalus; blindness, secondary to primary optic atrophy; quadriplegia, severe.

History

Background Information

Sally was the first of four children born to a 21-year-old mother. Records indicate she was apparently normal at birth. However, six months after delivery she was noted to have a hydrocephalus and has had in her young life frequent shunting problems. She has lived home since birth except for a short placement at the state school.

Sally's physical disabilities are considerable; thus, she requires total care by others; her mother has been primary caretaker. Sally's disabilities have restricted her interactions with other people and the environment; therefore, exposure to typical and necessary experiences needed for growth has not taken place. Sally has been extensively evaluated but has remained primarily homebound.

Educational History

In the past, she received one year of tutoring from the local school system. Sally had 15 months of workshop experience at the workshop for the blind under Vocational Rehabilitation which began in 1976 and ended in 1977, when she was discharged due to her inability to perform task. Home programming was made available from the Office of Mental Retardation from 1978 until 1979; Client Management and family continued this service until March 1979, which ended due to difficulties in the home.

At the age of 21, she no longer was eligible for Crippled Children Services, school programs, or programs for the visually handicapped. Previous to age 21, she had received minimal services from these programs.

Current Level of Functioning

At the time of her last testing, Sally was assessed to be functioning at the moderate range of mental retardation basically caused by environmental deprivation due to her extensive medical and physical limitations. She does not possess daily living skills. Sally's short-term auditory memory is poor, and she attempts to answer questions impulsively. She also needs frequent reassurance when attempting new tasks. Sally always cooperates and is eager to please, but when she begins to experience difficulty she will become frustrated. When frustrated she begins to demonstrate mannerisms such as sounds emanating from her mouth and head rolling. When she is confronted with a task or a situation she does not want to deal with, she will say, ''I've had enough of that,'' or fall asleep, instead of spending the time and energy necessary to resolve the problem.

Sally demonstrates good communication skills, but her receptive and expressive skills are not based upon extensive experiences with the environment. This lack of experience limits her comprehension of situations that are not based on concrete experiences.

Problems in Obtaining Needed Services

Day Program/Educational Service

Sally was not an appropriate candidate for a sheltered workshop environment due to lack of necessary skills needed to be eligible. Because of her limited abilities and lack of available services, she has been homebound. Welfare, the Office of Mental Retardation, the family, and later Client Management paid for home programming services for her from Spring 1978 until Spring 1979, which ended due to difficulties in the home.

The family for the most part has been the sole and primary caretaker for Sally with little if any support from the "system." Through the years they have developed a resentment towards the "system" for not assisting them in the needed support and services for their daughter. It appears that her family has adapted her physical management to the family life-style and that any alterations in the home routine have been met with resistance from the family. Consequently, Sally's parents felt that a home aide created an additional burden to the family since his/her presence interfered with the family's life-style. They felt that unless services such as day programming could be provided for outside the home, they would meet her needs solely on their own.

Housing

She continues to reside in her home with her family. The situation has improved considerably since her involvement in a day program. Three weeks of summer camp has allowed respite for the family for the past two summers. Currently, a respite program which could be provided to the family throughout the year on a regular basis is in the process of being developed.

Transportation

Transportation has always presented barriers for Sally and has in many ways kept her, and particularly her mother, confined to the home. Until recently, since access to commercial wheelchair transportation service was not available, it was necessary for her father to lift and carry her into the car. This has now become an impossible task due to her size. There is no public transportation in the region, and the only available wheelchair service to be contracted with was from another state at the cost of $30 a round trip. Taxi service was also sought, but it was found not to be a feasible alternative. Medicaid covers the cost of commercial service if used infrequently, but the service was needed on a daily basis to transport Sally to the day program. Welfare agreed to subsidize the cost for a 60-day period at $14 a round trip leaving the remaining cost to the family or another service provider.

The Regional Client Management Board agreed this past June that for Sally, and many other individuals who are developmentally disabled in the community and those returning from the institution, programming was being jeopardized due to the lack of a transportation system in the region. The Board endorsed the development of a transportation program by the Region Client Management in order to facilitate the transport of individuals to the Adult Day Program and the Sheltered Workshop in the region. Title XX is providing mileage reimbursement at 15¢ a mile per client from their home to the location they are deposited and $14 a day for Sally's wheelchair service with the rest of the van and driver's salary being funded by the Client Management budget.

Medical Services

Access to local medical services has always been readily available to Sally. However, services from special programs such as Crippled Children Services and New Hampshire Services for the Visually Handicapped were terminated when she turned 21 years old due to eligibility criteria. There are no special medical services readily available for adults in this state who are as physically handicapped as she is. Visiting Nurses Services are available, but their services in the region are limited.

Generic Services

Transportation has been and is one of the major limiting factors in integrating into community services. Until recently, her total environment evolved around her home and family. Attempts have been made to use recreational services; however, lack of community awareness has not facilitated her involvement.

A real Case Management dilemma without community supports in place and accessible—especially in rural areas.

CLIENT MANAGEMENT CASE STUDY #3
BETTY – A 12-YEAR-OLD FEMALE

Reason for Referral: Deinstitutionalization from the state school (after 10 years of residency)

Diagnosis: Profound mental retardation with other conditions (unspecified), no genetic mechanism present; microcephaly, secondary; no apparent sensory impairment; no speech; major motor seizures; no psychiatric in,pairment present; spasticity; quadriplegia, moderate.

History

Family Background

Betty was the second of two known children born to a young mother whose first pregnancy ended in a miscarriage. Her parents are divorced. According to the divorce decree, the father has custody, and the parents are co-legal guardians. Her father remarried and resides in New Hampshire. He is self-employed. Her stepmother is a professional. There have been no children from this marriage. Betty's oldest brother is a freshman in high school, lives with his father, and is in good health. Her father visited once in 1977; he reports that Betty recognizes him. At last report, her mother had remarried; her last known address is another state where she is employed as a cosmetic salesperson. She visits Betty regularly. No vacations with family are recorded.

Educational History

Betty has not received any educational services until this past year. She currently is enrolled in a Readiness Class for three hours a day, for four days a week.

Medical Background

Her last physical examination was done in 1978. She has no allergies. She has a major motor seizure disorder and is observed as having flash-type seizures, a series of six or eight, three or four times a month. She is receiving phenobarbital grains, one-half twice a day, for seizure control. She is moderate spastic quadriplegic. She is out of bed in a wheelchair or positioned in a bean bag. She has no feeding skills. She is fully fed a ground diet. She has no bathing or dressing skills and is incontinent with occasional problems with constipation. She needs complete care with oral hygiene. Betty is nonverbal, and her vision is impaired by Alternating Estotropia and Bilateral Nystagmus. Her hearing is said to be adequate.

Current Status

Level of Functioning

At the time of her last developmental assessment, Betty was found to be functioning at the developmental levels of 9-12 months in feeding, play, and receptive language skills; 4-8 months in motor skills (with splinter skills at higher levels); and 1-3 months in expressive language skills.

Betty is quite alert and responsive to her environment. She is currently dependent on others for her feeding, dressing, toileting, and grooming care. She cooperates when being dressed, by extending her arm. She is responsive to social stimulation. She smiles at others and follows moving persons with her head and eyes; she also appears to recognize significant adults in her life.

She demonstrates some language development, identifies and shows functions of objects. She also attempts to imitate motor behavior with prompting. Betty indicates wants by gestures, shaking her head, and facial expressions.

Her level of functioning is somewhat restricted by her generalized spasticity; however, she does demonstrate limited use of her right hand and arm. Her current level of adaptive behavior functioning is within the profound range of mental retardation.

Present Residence and Future Enrollment

As a resident of the state school, Betty is limited in actual services provided to her. Ideally, the Children's Team has requested that she be an active client, receiving all the services provided by the specialist who evaluated her. However, due to limited resources and staff, the yearly evaluations are the extent of the services provided. For the first time this year, she is receiving minimal educational programming.

Betty has been placed on active status for community placement. Arrangements have been made for her enrollment in a development center.

Here, she will receive educational programming and speech, physical, and occupational therapy. The center's philosophy is based on the principle of development and team approach to services, regardless of the severity of the individuals' handicaps. The proposal plan regards her present level of functioning as a starting point and will attempt to increase her level of functioning in all areas of development by encouraging progress along a normal developmental sequence.

Results of Programming

Progress reports indicate from the stimulation and experiences being provided through the Educational Department Readiness Class that Betty is definitely acquiring new skills and has made gains in cognitive and social development. The center's staff feels that with total programming and community placement in a foster home, Betty will demonstrate substantial gains. Presently it is difficult to predict, due to her limited services and institutional setting which are not conducive to social responsiveness and intellectual growth.

Report on Community Placement Status

Upon review of 18 state school residents, Betty was identified as one of six individuals from a region whose needs could be met in the community. This choice was discussed with various staff members at the school as well as professionals employed by a development center and other community agencies.

Betty's teacher at the state school visited the development center and agreed it was an appropriate educational setting. The program coordinator for the development center previously observed Betty while at the state school and he also felt that the development center could provide an appropriate educational program, as well as necessary support services: speech therapy, physical therapy, and occupational therapy.

Attempts were made by Client Management to locate an appropriate foster home for Betty. A licensed foster home demonstrated much interest in her and was eager to pursue placement within their home.

Previous to locating appropriate services for Betty, several attempts were made to discuss community placement with her father. It was not until March 1979 that her father agreed to meet with me and visit the development center. The following community alternatives were discussed with him and his wife.

Community Placement

Services	Service Provider
Housing	Licensed foster home
Day program	Development center
Speech therapy	Development center
Physical therapy	Development center
Occupational therapy	Development center
Yearly audiological/vision screening	Development center
Medical services:	Local pediatrician
(seizure monitoring)	Visiting Nurses Association
(immunization update)	Crippled Children's Seizure Clinic
Lab work	Clinic
Dental services	Local dentist
Socialization/recreation	Companionship Project
	Town Recreation
	Summer Camp
Transportation	Title XX — vendor service

They also observed classes at the development center and spoke to staff.

Betty's father did not feel that his daughter would benefit from community placement at this time. He felt that she appeared content in her current placement and that the services being provided her were sufficient.

He and his wife stated that because Client Management could not guarantee a successful placement and substantial developmental gains in her current skill level, he could not support this effort. He also mentioned that he had consulted his family physician on this matter and that the physician agreed that community placement was not appropriate.

I was disappointed by his decision. I strongly believe that Betty could have benefited substantially from community placement. As of that decision date, she will be put on inactive status indefinitely. However, her father did agree that I should maintain future contact in case he should reconsider.

General Problems in Obtaining Necessary Services Inherent
in Case Management

Housing

Currently in this region there are no housing alternatives for severely handicapped individuals whose families cannot provide care in their own home. Even for those who can, there are minimal, if any, supports to the family, e.g., respite care.

This worker discovered that there were no easily accessible listings of existing licensed foster homes which may be able to provide a home to severely involved individuals. Welfare was resistant in releasing names of foster homes for fear of competition in a scarce commodity, especially since Client Management was willing to pay an additional stipend and provide support to a foster home which was willing to accept a Client Management client.

Welfare's only involvement with this case was to provide names of existing licensed homes and agreed to the process for a home which the client manager may have located in attempting to obtain foster care. The client manager sent out approximately 100 letters and received approximately ten responses. Out of the ten, only four individuals showed any real interest. The client manager visited each of the homes and chose one as a viable alternative.

Medical/Dental Services

Medical and dental services are not easily acquired for individuals who are developmentally disabled. Only a limited number of medical professionals are available who are willing and/or trained to deal with the individual who is developmentally impaired. Adding to this difficulty is the resistance of many physicians to take on Medicaid recipients as clients. However, Visiting Nurses Association will monitor the individual's general health in the home on a monthly basis if specified by physician. Also, Crippled Children's Seizure Clinic offers a wide range of medical services to children up to the age of 21.

Client Management has attempted to recruit medical and dental services on an individual client basis. Usually, arrangements are made through phone, letter, and personal contact with the client manager. Currently, this process has proved successful for the small numbers of individuals for which the client manager needed to recruit services. However, there is concern that this method may no longer be effective when large numbers of individuals are returned from the state school to the community.

On a larger scale, the client manager, in conjunction with other service brokers from Welfare, Mental Health and Education, attempted to develop a listing for reference purposes of medical and dental professionals who were willing to accept as clients individuals who are developmentally disabled. Many local doctors and dentists who were contacted refused to allow their names to be listed.

Educational Services

Arrangements are made, through the client manager, to have clients attend the development center. The public schools in this region do not have classes for individuals who are functioning at the profound/severe range of retardation. The public school is ultimately responsible for seeing that the educational services are provided. It is also responsible for the cost and development of the individual service plan.

The cost of the program for a client is $6,500 a year which also includes physical therapy, speech therapy, and occupational therapy services. Fortunately, in specific cases, appropriate educational services are available in the region.

Generic Services

Integrating the client into generic agencies which serve the general public such as local recreation groups at this time has proved difficult to attain. Much of the resistance stems from lack of awareness and unnecessary concerns on the part of the community. With time, the development of community education programs, and support to the generic agency, access to these services will be attained more easily.

Transportation

Transportation to and from educational services is the responsibility of the public schools. Transportation to other services is provided by foster family or another private party; mileage (in some cases) is paid for by Welfare.

Transportation is a major problem for most clients. However, being nonambulatory and needing a vehicle which can accommodate a wheelchair have made many conventional services (such as a private cars and/or a taxi service) inaccessible.

Financial Assistance

A particular client could be eligible for the following financial assistance.

   *A) SSI, Medicaid Special Education, and Welfare
   *B) Client Management Funds

The following is a breakdown of financial responsibility for various services:

Housing	Both Welfare & Case Management (* & **)
Foster home	**
Respite care	
Medical services	*
Dental services	**
Evaluations	*
Recreation	**
Therapy	*
Transportation	**

All the services mentioned are arranged for clients by the client manager. If the family agrees to community placement, a total individual service plan is developed by the client manager in coordination with the other service providers responsible for providing services to the client.

Chapter 12

MENTAL HEALTH PROGRAMS

Dawn Nelson, M.Ed.

CLIENT MANAGEMENT CASE STUDY #1
H. – A 35-YEAR-OLD MALE

H. is a 35-year-old, divorced, Catholic male who was referred to the Mental Health Center upon discharge from a state hospital following a one-year admission. Recommendation from the hospital was simply for follow-up care and daytime activities, as client was to live with his father who had recently bought a house specifically so that H. could live with him.

Past History

H. was the sixth of eight children. The father was a lumberjack and an alcoholic who had a tendency, while intoxicated, to abuse physically his wife and children. The mother was a domineering and overprotective person who worked in a hatchery.

H. has a long history of medical problems, dating back to age 11 months, when he apparently had a brain hemorrhage, after which he reportedly began "twitching uncontrollably." He was first diagnosed at age 14 as having a seizure disorder although there is a possibility that this condition existed before that.

School performance was always poor. The client attended school through the eighth grade. Social interactions were limited; the client had few friends and kept pretty much to himself.

After leaving school, H. worked at odd jobs for several years. At age 17 H.'s parents were divorced (the mother filed because the father was apparently dating other women). H. went to live with his father, while the other seven children lived with the mother.

It was also at age 17 that H. began working in a factory. He worked there steadily for two years. During this period of time H.'s seizures reportedly occurred frequently, but this was apparently not so problematic that it prohibited him from working largely because his boss was "understanding," and he worked with "the girl next door," who would watch over him to some extent.

At age 19, H. married "the girl next door." There was, according to this client, some discord in the marriage since the client preferred a life centered around the house, and his wife was more social, preferring to go out and to be active.

At age 20, the client accidentally ran into a telephone pole while playing baseball and hit his head. As a result of this accident, seizures became more severe and frequent, his short-term memory was impaired, and the client became delusional.

The client was no longer able to maintain his job (due to the seizures and short-term memory impairment) and began receiving disability payments at this time.

For the following five years, the client spent most of his time at home. He has three children, the first of whom was born before the accident, and the second two were born after he became disabled. H. was isolated, for the most part, from social interactions except with his wife, children, mother, father, and stepfather during this time.

H. became increasingly more delusional and was first hospitalized for psychiatric reasons at age 25 for a period of 30 days. Since that time, H. has had repeated and lengthy hospitalizations.

At age 29, H. and his wife were divorced. (The divorce was initiated by his wife, and she remarried shortly thereafter.) H. was apparently particularly disturbed about leaving his children.

H. rented an apartment after the divorce, which he lived in while not in the hospital. Concern was expressed by his parents over the acceptability of H. living independently considering his seizures and his inability to take his medication regularly due to his memory difficulties. However, this client was adamant at this time about maintaining this living arrangement since he wanted to live in a way which was conducive to maintaining contact with his children.

At age 34, while in his apartment, a fire started in an overstuffed chair. How this fire started was unclear. It was clear that it was unintentional and probably the result of H. either smoking or ironing, having a seizure or forgetting about what he was doing, and having the hot object ignite the chair. He was not badly hurt, and the fire was extinguished. At this time, H. was again hospitalized largely because of pressure from his family who said that he was unable to live independently and was a danger to himself.

H. was then hospitalized for a year. During this time, H. was found to have an unusual problem with his blood; a high serum iron content. Apparently the only treatment for this condition is removing blood from the individual's body on a regular basis, and if this is not done, the person's life is in eventual danger. H.'s paranoid delusions have continued to exist since the baseball accident at age 20, and, despite repeated explanations regarding the iron in his blood, he continues to suspect that efforts to remove blood are meant to kill him eventually. The concept of the blood replacing itself in his body is difficult for him, as is it difficult for him to trust the explanations of others in relationship to this.

Initial Contact with Mental Health Center

During this hospitalization, H.'s father (whose health was failing by this time) decided to buy a house so that H. could live with him. After being hospitalized for one year, H. was discharged to live with his father and to attend programs at the mental health center.

H. immediately began attending programs at the mental health center. He was found by us to be, on one hand, an intelligent and creative individual with a great deal of pride and insistence on being his own person. On the other hand, he was a person with extensive limitations, not all of which he easily accepted (particularly the limitations imposed on what he could do by his short-term memory difficulty and the possibility of a seizure at any time). He was also a person whose trust in the word of others was precarious and in whom there was an almost constant delusion (which primarily centered around the idea that the persons were not really treating his medical condition but were trying to kill him).

Most striking was his work in the woodshop. He was able to make his own patterns for building small cabinets, etc., on his own initiative, and to solve problems related to building them independently. His work was of impeccable quality. (However, he was never satisfied with his work.)

Additionally, he did seem to begin to develop some degree of trust in two staff members, both of whom were willing to let him try to find solutions to his problems rather than telling him that he wasn't able to do so.

Two weeks after discharge from the hospital, H.'s father died.

Case Management

At this point, it became clear that facilitating adequate and desirable housing for H. was a central treatment and case management goal. What became more clear over the following weeks was that treatment and case management with this client were so closely intertwined that they were difficult to separate.

H.'s mother stated that he could stay with her on a short-term basis until adequate housing was found. H. was agreeable to this. Since there were no other alternatives available and since everyone agreed that H.'s continuing to live independently in the father's house was not desirable, we decided that this was the most viable option.

In retrospect, what was not spelled out clearly enough was the difficulty in finding a living situation that was desirable, available, and acceptable to all involved.

H. maintained that he wanted to and was able to live independently. He presented elaborate and sound plans for monitoring his medication, considering carefully the limitations of his memory. It seemed that his main reason for living independently was to have a place suitable for visits from his children, with whom it seemed vitally important to H. to maintain contact.

His mother (who was now very much in the picture) maintained that H. was unable to live independently, that we could all see from the last experience how dangerous this was. Furthermore, she maintained that we were to find a place for him to live and to do it quickly as she could not have H. at her house for long. (She stated that her new marriage was in jeopardy due to the stress H. caused at home.)

It became clear to us that, regardless of the desirability or lack thereof of a group home or independent living to either H. or his mother, we were in the middle of a family fight, a position not conducive to problem solving.

The first meeting with H. with his mother present was held several weeks later. Both H. and his mother held their stances firmly during this meeting. The mental health center firmly stated the following: (1) (to H. in the presence of his mother) that we were seriously concerned about the safety of his living independently, but that we had no right to stop him if this was his choice, and that we would try to help him in any way we could if he chose to pursue this; (2) (to the mother, in the presence of H.) that we saw the choice as being between them, that we could give both of them information about group homes and/or get them connected with a welfare worker who had more information than we did about group homes on a statewide basis, but that we could not, based on the disagreement between them, make contacts to place H. in a group home because H. stated that this was unacceptable to him. Furthermore, we made it clear to both of them that, should the mother's choice be to ask H. to leave her house, we had no solution to alternative living situations.

During the following several months there was a great deal of activity, but no changes.

H. was encouraged to look into apartment prices and to consider the possibility of living with a roommate. This was an angering process to him, as he realized that the expense was too great for him to afford on disability payments. His tendency was to blame all involved with his being hospitalized after the fire (stating that this hospitalization was what caused him to lose his old apartment) rather than to consider that this physical limitation may influence his ability to live independently.

H. was referred to Vocational Rehabilitation and did follow-up on the interview there. He was basically told by Voc. Rehab. that they could not work with him towards his chosen vocation as a carpenter or handyman, not because of his lack of ability, but because they would not be able to place him due to his memory and seizure difficulties. (The risk to an employer would be too great.)

H. spent time (at his mother's request) at two group homes in our catchment area. In one home there was no space and H. did not like it, and in the other case H. was found to be unacceptable due to his being much more able, in many ways, than the other residents.

Welfare was contacted by our agency, and a listing of group homes in the state was given to H. and his mother. The mother was to be the primary person to make the contacts if her hope was to place H. in a group home, which she did. The difficulties in finding an adequate placement became apparent to her through this process, and while it did not dispel her anger at or her demand on the social service agencies involved, it did seem to give her a more realistic perspective of what was possible.

Difficulties were found by either H. or his mother with each of the few group homes in which there were openings.

The mental health center finally suggested that if nothing available was acceptable, maybe serious consideration needed to be given to independent living. It was at this point that H. finally agreed that he probably could not handle an apartment. He clearly understood that living with his mother was not an option since there had been considerable tension between them during his stay. H., his mother, and the mental health center were now in more agreement than ever before about what needed to be done; a sheltered living situation needed to be located which offered H. maximum independence and integrity, which was affordable, and where productive use of his time could be made, either within the living situation or without.

All parties involved then began this search. An independent group home was finally located by the mental health center, in which the owner was in need of a general handyman and helper. This owner was excited about the prospect of a resident of the home helping out in this way and was willing to negotiate what fee to pay for this service. While disability payments did not completely cover the cost of living in this home, the difference could easily be made up by payments for H.'s services. The need for his help seemed to enhance the client's sense of worth but not to put him in a highly dangerous position due to his seizures or memory difficulty, since a responsible person would be nearby.

At this time, the mental health center realized the importance of not taking responsibility for placement, but rather to work as a facilitator. H. and his mother were notified of this possibility and given a name and number to call. The owner of the home was informed about the client and his situation. H. made the contact and went for a visit.

The owner liked the client and was willing to accept him. The client found the situation to be acceptable. The client's mother found the situation to be acceptable but wanted the owner to take total responsibility for all aspects of the client's life. The mother and owner began arguing about who would do what.

This group home was outside of the catchment area, but a decision was made that to ensure a successful transition, case management responsibilities should continue for 6 months.

The case manager clinically assessed the situation, and a decision was made that, at this time, mother and owner were unable to resolve their differences. If difficulties between the two of them could not be resolved, the placement would be in jeopardy, and we knew of no other options.

The case manager spoke with the mother and notified her of our concern over the possibility of the placement falling through because of the squabbling between the owner and her. The case manager reiterated to the mother that we knew of no other options.

The case manager then contacted the owner of the group home. The owner was supported by the case manager when she stated that she couldn't be held responsible for every aspect of each resident's life and that she simply needed to set limits somewhere.

An appointment had already been set up for H. at the local community mental health center. Telephone contact had been made, and records had been sent. The argument between the owner and the mother had revolved around who was to be responsible for insuring that H.'s medical treatment was taken care of. Contact needed to be made with a good physician in the area to which he was moving, and transportation needed to be arranged. With all of the changes, H. was becoming more delusional, especially about the bleeding that needed to be done. The local mental health center was not, as yet, involved, and no alliance between them and the client had been established.

The case manager contacted a local physician for help in locating a good physician in the new area, then contacted the new physician, arranged for an appointment and for the medical history to be transferred, and described the difficulties of client care for the medical condition as we saw it. The case manager spoke with the owner of the group home who agreed to take the client to the physician if there were no complications.

The case manager then decided that, until an alliance was developed with the local mental health center, the client was more comfortable in his new surroundings, and the tension regarding the uncertainties of this change diminished, it would be important for her to maintain contact with the client.

The case manager visited the client on a weekly basis in the group home for a period of about two months. During these visits she saw her role as being primarily to reality test with him about the current happenings in his life and to monitor his ability to adapt to the changes. These visits seemed to reassure the client adequately.

The visits were discontinued about 3 months ago. Follow-up contact will be made by her with the mental health center in that area. She will pay one final visit to the client to insure that things are going smoothly, and the case will be closed.

CLIENT MANAGEMENT CASE STUDY #2
M. – A 63-YEAR-OLD FEMALE

The client is a 63-year-old, white, protestant, married woman who was recently referred to the mental health center from the state hospital where she had been receiving treatment for two months.

The client and her husband have apparently been happily married and continue to seem quite dedicated to each other. They have two adult children, both of whom live in this catchment area and are willing to continue to be involved with their parents. (The son has temporary guardianship of his mother and has applied for permanent guardianship.)

The couple have spent much of their life in the Chicago area. It was at the time of the client's admission to the hospital that they were planning to move back to New England. The decision for this move was based on: (1) the client showing early signs of senility, (2) the husband's health failing, and, as a result of these factors, (3) wanting to live closer to their children, in case anything should happen to one or the other.

Apparently both the client and her husband have led active and fulfilling lives. About four years ago the wife started having increased difficulty with her short-term memory and has required more careful supervision by her husband with daily living activities. At the same time, the husband began having difficulty with his heart.

In April of this year the two of them came to this area to visit their children and to find a place to live. It was during this visit that the client decompensated (became severely confused, disoriented × 3, suspicious of others, incoherent, and showed severely impaired judgment) and, at the same time, the husband suffered a severe heart attack. The husband was hospitalized for medical reasons; the wife was hospitalized for psychiatric reasons.

The husband, upon recovery from the heart attack went back to Chicago with his son and sold the house there. A trailer was purchased by him at a trailer park close to the son's home. The client was stabilized with medication and, upon discharge from the hospital, moved directly into this trailer with her husband.

Referral to Mental Health Center and Case Management

The client (and her husband) were evaluated by the mental health center within a week after discharge. It was decided that the client needed considerable supervision; she tends to forget what she is doing and has a tendency not to eat adequately since her mind wanders. While her husband was able and willing to do this, the strain it placed on him to do it on a full-time basis seemed to jeopardize his health further.

Neither the client nor the husband has support systems in this area other than their family. Both children work and have their own families, so the extent to which they can lend support is limited by their circumstances.

The client was referred to the Day Treatment Program: (1) to encourage client to remain as active as possible, (2) to monitor medication and eating to some extent, and (3) to give husband the respite he needs for his own health.

The Elderly Services worker from this agency was contacted by the case manager, met with the husband, and offered him assistance in eliciting support for him in the following forms: (1) receiving financial assistance from Welfare to get a homemaker to help with the housework, (2) becoming involved, with his wife, in a meal program at a local senior center, and (3) having the Welcome Wagon visit. The husband agreed to all of the forms of support. The Elderly Services worker called the various service providers, explained the circumstances to them, and arranged for services to be provided.

The son was then contacted and will be in soon to meet with the case manager. The purpose of this meeting will be: (1) to clarify the role the mental health center is assuming in relationship to his parents, (2) to clarify the extent to which he is willing to be involved (particularly if his father's health should fail), (3) to develop, with him, a plan for insuring that his mother receives adequate care and supervision in the least restrictive setting should his father become unable, for whatever reason, to continue caring for her, and (4) to offer our continued assistance to both him and his parents in whatever way is possible.

At this time the client is attending the Day Program three days per week, and, while the senility will not go away, she seems to be in good spirits, to be making new friends, to eat well while she is here, and to be beginning to involve herself in some crafts activities (for the first time in four years).

The husband is becoming involved at the senior center, both with and without his wife. Homemaker services are beginning.

The case will require continued monitoring of wife, husband, and the adequacy of the support systems relative to changes in each of their conditions.

CLIENT MANAGEMENT CASE STUDY #3
A. – A 48-YEAR-OLD FEMALE

A. is a 48-year-old, divorced, Catholic female who was the seventh of ten children. She has a high school education, was married at age 19, and is the mother of eight children (current ages are 9 to 25).

On different occasions members of the community in which this family has lived for many years have described a similar picture and sentiment for this family. Basically the description is of a healthy and active family, who were involved in the community while the children were small and were generally well liked and respected. Most often the comments are followed by "that poor family!"

Apparently, over the years, the husband began drinking heavily and became abusive. The client seemed eventually to become unable to set limits on either her husband's or children's behavior. After 22 years of marriage, the client and her husband were divorced.

Psychiatric History

A.'s first contact with psychiatric professionals occurred at about the time when client had became religiously involved to psychotic proportions and was hospitalized at a private hospital for two weeks. Following this, she was able to return home to her children, and there was no follow-up care.

She was again hospitalized in 1974 after becoming confused, disorganized, and paranoid. This time, she had divided her house into compartments for good and evil and the children into bad and good. She was followed in supportive therapy on a monthly basis after this hospitalization.

Her third hospitalization (again the client was psychotic) was in 1976. It was from this hospitalization that she was referred to the mental health center.

Initial Treatment

Upon referral client was not psychotic, was working on a part-time basis as a nurses aide (and apparently was a valued worker at the nursing home in which she worked), had a close personal relationship with a sister who lived nearby, and had five of her eight children living at home. She seemed to continue to have difficulty in maintaining order in her house with the five remaining children.

It was decided that the client was in greatest need of support on an ongoing basis and help in limit setting as well as ongoing monitoring of medication. She was referred to an ongoing women's support group and was to meet with a nurse on a regular basis to follow medication, and to get some help in limit setting.

This treatment program was effective for a period of about two years. A. seemed to be able to maintain her work and her household but continued to require considerable support and assistance in doing so. Her support systems included: (1) the mental health center, (2) Welfare (who helped with financial support), and (3) her sister, who was also divorced and with whom client maintained telephone contact several times each day.

During the summer of 1978, the stress at home with the children being older, more difficult to manage, and home for summer vacation became more than A. could handle. This marked the beginning of her most recent regression.

Case Management

At this time Welfare was contacted, and temporary foster homes were located for the two youngest children.

The client was assessed, and it was determined that she was not able to continue managing the household, even with the two youngest children absent. The one child who would be able to assist in this effort was in the armed forces and was not to be discharged for three months.

It was the joint opinion of the staff and the client that having this son home at this time was the preferable solution. The son was contacted and stated that he would be happy to do this. The son's commanding officer was contacted and was instrumental in assisting the mental health center in securing an early discharge for her son.

Within four days from when it became apparent that client was unable to manage, the younger children were removed from the home, and the most responsible son was brought home from the service.

The client contacted her boss at work, who was willing to give her a leave of absence from her job (which she was unable to handle at this time).

She began attending the Day Treatment Program at the mental health center to decrease isolation and potential of further regression.

By the end of the summer the client had recompensated to the extent that her son was able to return home. (The younger children were back in school, and the case manager maintained contact with the guidance counselor at the younger children's school.) A. was not yet able to return to work.

About one month thereafter, the client's sister died unexpectedly. Again she became depressed and was less able to function.

The family was again under stress. The older children at home were beginning to get into trouble with the police. The younger children were showing signs of stress at school. Family therapy did not seem to offer an adequate solution to the current situation because the children were not willing to participate at this time.

The case manager then escalated liaison efforts with the police and the school, seeing her role as being primarily to clarify any misunderstandings they might have about the client's current conditions, as well as to serve as a consultant to these persons to find ways in which they might deal with the children. This contact seemed to alleviate a great deal of the anxiety that the police and counselor were feeling and to help them to be more sensitive in their dealings with the children, and the children seemed to settle down somewhat as a result of this.

The client continued to attend the program on a daily basis and over a period of several months seemed to be again gaining some strength.

Then again, just as she seemed to be making some improvements, the bottom fell out from under her when one of her sons developed cancer. At about the same time, the client developed a medical difficulty in her arm which limited her movement (and would limit the possibility of her eventually returning to work at the nursing home).

All persons associated with members of this family were notified. The son was operated on, apparently successfully.

The client, during the interim, again became more depressed. However, over the following four months, she continued to attend the program regularly and continued to improve.

At this time A. decided that she could not return to her job at the nursing home due to the problem with her arm. Instead she took a job through a temporary employment agency to test out her ability to return to work. She found that she was ready to begin working again.

Competing in the open market for a job seemed to hold the potential of causing significant stress. At the same time, Vocational Rehabilitation seemed inappropriate because job training was not really needed at this time. CETA was seen as a more viable option and was contacted.

The client began working for CETA several months ago. Her principal work seems to revolve around gathering data for human service agencies, and she has a great deal of contact with people. She seems to enjoy it and be good at it.

She continues to have some difficulty setting limits with her children, but life at home is as steady as it has ever been.

The client continues to have contact with the mental health center on a regular basis for support, monitoring, medication, and for help in limit setting. She is currently coming in on a biweekly basis for one hour.

Chapter 13

WELFARE PROGRAMS

Thomas Salatiello, M.S.W.

CLIENT MANAGEMENT CASE STUDY #1
SARAH – AN 80-YEAR-OLD FEMALE

Sarah became known to the Division of Welfare in 1974 at the age of 75. She was alone after her husband's death and found adjustment to life extremely difficult. Indications from the client were that her husband had handled all household matters and had been very protective of her. As a result, she felt incapable of maintaining an independent living situation. An effort was made to find a live-in companion; but after several interviews, the client rejected this possibility as inappropriate.

Sarah moved to a three-room, first floor apartment a short distance from her previous home. One of her neighbors apparently befriended her and, within a short time, ridiculed her to others. She told Sarah that none of the neighbors liked her. This caused Sarah more unhappiness, and she began to withdraw from all social contacts. She became extremely depressed, a condition later diagnosed as chronic depression with chronic brain syndrome. Another striking factor at this time was her deteriorating physical condition due to improper eating habits. Sarah's weight dropped to 85 pounds.

The social worker arranged for Sarah to have a physical examination, and a referral was made to the Mental Health Clinic. Records state that although she tried to act and relate confidently, it was obvious that she was disoriented and lethargic. Contact with the Mental Health Agency was discontinued at her request.

In conjunction with the direct services provided by the Division of Welfare, the services of a homemaker and nurse were enlisted. Daily meals from the Meals on Wheels Program were provided, and minimal assistance from a neighbor was authorized through Title XX to provide night and weekend coverage of meal preparation. Although Sarah was having difficulty managing her money, the suggestion of obtaining a protective payee to manage her finances and assure the payment of her bills was unacceptable to her.

Records indicate that despite attempts to assure Sarah that she would be cared for in her apartment, she repeatedly expressed concern that she would be placed in an institution. Physical belongings, in particular her cat and dog, became very important to her; and she became unwilling to leave her apartment for any reason. Her physical condition continued to deteriorate, and despite efforts to improve her nutrition the client persisted in sporadic eating habits. Direct services continued, and Title XX Adult In Home Day Care was authorized in 1976 to provide meal preparation, shopping, and supervision of her personal care routines throughout the entire week. After the establishment of a positive relationship between Sarah and her day care provider, a dependency developed that limited Sarah's willingness to express her needs. Her fear of losing her provider's attentions added complications to the client/provider relationship.

In early 1977, the addition of a Senior Companion was added to Sarah's case planning. The primary function of a companion is to provide another elderly person with a peer relationship that is supportive. Sarah was particularly responsive to this service as she had lost contact with former friends, and this peer relationship provided areas of mutual interest. This service is unique in that the companion does not provide household services. She is able, therefore, to spend time talking with the client, playing Scrabble, and walking the dog.

The goal in this case continues to be community-based care. The direct services of Individual and Family Adjustment as well as Adult In Home Day Care, a paid service, are being provided by the Division of Welfare. In conjunction, the Community Health Agency is providing homemaking and nursing services. Meals on Wheels are delivered daily, and the Senior Companion continues to visit. There continues to be concern over finances, but Sarah is reluctant to question her provider, whom she delegated to pay bills and make purchases. As the provider gives Sarah no receipts, she is unable to determine her exact expenses. Sarah becomes disturbed that she is unable to save any money after her monthly utilities and food bills have been paid. Sarah is unwilling to mention this to her provider as she feels any indication of a lack of trust will result in her rejection. This fear is reinforced by the defensive behavior exhibited by the provider when questioned. Suggestions by the social worker that she have a third party as a protective payee continue to be rejected, and she will in no way allow anyone to question the provider.

This is clearly a manipulative situation. However, since Sarah's physical and emotional dependency on her provider and her tendency to become seriously depressed remain, it has been decided to allow the situation to remain as it is for the present.

Overall, this is a case which demonstrates inter-agency involvement in keeping an 80-year-old individual functioning in her own environment. Frequent conversations between the social worker and the visiting nurse, as well as occasional meetings which include the homemakers, keep those involved aware of changes in behavior and allow for the reassessment of needs. In addition to this, the social worker meets weekly with the Senior Companion who also provides input. The services of the In Home Day Care provider are monitored by both the social worker and visiting nurse. Without community services, it is unlikely that Sarah could maintain herself, and an institutional placement would be necessary.

CLIENT MANAGEMENT CASE STUDY #2
EMILY – A 24-YEAR-OLD FEMALE

Emily, a 24-year-old woman with cerebral palsy who is confined to a wheelchair, wanted to move from her parents' home into her own apartment. Emily also wanted her 32-year-old sister, Liz, to share the apartment with her. Liz had always helped care for Emily in their parents' home and was agreeable to try independent living. Although she was borderline mentally retarded, she could help Emily with personal care and household chores.

Many social agencies combined efforts in the process of arranging independent living for Liz and Emily. Both women were directly involved in the location of a suitable apartment. They checked advertisements and called landlords. As Emily had difficulty getting around, Liz and the Welfare social worker would look at the apartment; and if it seemed appropriate, Emily would then go to see it. Emily and Liz made the final decision in choosing their apartment and made arrangements with the landlord with minimal social worker involvement.

The next step was to furnish the apartment and have Emily and Liz move in. The women had some furniture of their own but other necessary items were supplemented by their family, Community Action, and City Welfare. As a participant in the sheltered workshop, Emily was able to borrow their van, driver, and a few employees to help with the moving process.

Once in their apartment, the women needed to supplement their incomes to meet their new expenses. Emily was already receiving SSI and State Welfare disability benefits. Liz had applied for assistance, but she had not yet been accepted. "Special needs" money was obtained from State Welfare to pay for the security deposit and telephone installation. Title XX social service funds were authorized to pay Liz for caring for Emily. City Welfare provided a food voucher, and an application for food stamps was completed.

Just prior to the women's move, all involved community agencies met to coordinate a case plan and assign tasks. This meeting included personnel from the sheltered workshop, State Welfare, Community Action, the senior center, Information and Referral, and the case manager for Belknap County. Each agency offered support to Liz and Emily in making their transition to independent living a positive experience. Their major problems were discussed, and a coordinated effort evolved to support their new-found independence.

Emily would continue to attend the sheltered workshop, and their van would provide her transportation to and from work. Other transportation problems for Emily such as doctor's visits and necessary errands would be provided by the workshop and Information and Referral volunteers. The case manager would be involved with visits involving great distance. The Community Action Program agreed to look into the possibility of a ramp for the apartment. The senior center wished to include Liz in their volunteer program one day a week to help her develop her own independence and become a participating member of the community. The case manager was available for counseling. The State Welfare social worker coordinated services and provided budget and supportive counseling when needed.

Emily and Liz have been living independently for about eight months. Last month they changed apartments as they had had some conflicts with the elderly ladies in their first apartment house. They located the apartment themselves and moved with the help of Community Action, City Welfare, and their father. Liz was accepted for disability benefits and still continues to receive Title XX funding for caring for her sister. The Community Health Agency is now seeing Emily once a week at her doctor's recommendation. She continues to attend the sheltered workshop. Both women receive counseling from the local Mental Health Center as they work through personal problems and deal with the pressures of their new independence.

It is possible that Emily and Liz may decide to move to a sheltered living arrangement, such as a shared home. The responsibilities involved with living on their own sometimes seem too great for them to cope with, given their limitations; however, community support systems are in place. Liz and Emily have had the opportunity to decide for themselves whether living independently is the best choice for them.

CLIENT MANAGEMENT CASE STUDY #3
MR. G. – A 70-YEAR-OLD MALE, MRS. G. – A 59-YEAR-OLD FEMALE, AND MS. H. – A 40-YEAR-OLD FEMALE

A referral was received from the local visiting nurse association revealing the multi-problemmed situation of Mr. and Mrs. G. and Ms. H.

Mr. G., a man in his seventies, was bedridden. He was cared for by his wife, a retarded woman in her late fifties, and a woman placed with the G.s as a domestic, who was also retarded. Both women had been residents of a state school for the retarded for a number of years.

The G.s and Ms. H. had been residing on the second floor of a house owned by Mr. G.'s nephew and had functioned reasonably well as a family unit. However, Mr. G.'s health deteriorated to the point where he became bedridden and unable to direct the affairs of the household. Beyond the evident need for a nursing home placement for Mr. G., it was also ascertained that the two women would require ongoing assistance to enable them to function adequately in the community. Although the women had to some extent held things together during Mr. G.'s deterioration, they lacked transportation, adequate housekeeping skills, money management capabilities, as well as food shopping and preparation skills.

The clients' residence was located eight miles from town. Mr. G.'s nephew, knowing that his uncle would soon be placed in a nursing home, withdrew from all involvement with the women and requested that they be relocated.

Mr. G. required an immediate nursing home placement. Finding a vacant bed in a local facility was most difficult as there had been a chronic shortage of nursing home beds in the area.

The ladiès, however, were relocated in a second floor apartment approximately 1-½ miles from town. The apartment was spacious, the rent reasonable, and, as time passed, the landlord and his wife were found to be an invaluable support system. Mr. G.'s nursing home was about ten miles from the ladies' apartment. Although Mrs. G. was unable to see her husband as frequently as she wanted, arrangements were made for her to visit her husband on a regular basis. On these visits she was also able to spend time speaking with the nursing home social worker.

As the alternatives for Mr. G.'s placement were chosen, concentration turned toward finalizing community plans for Mrs. G. and Ms. H. Mrs. G. met each suggestion with resistance as her ability to understand the scope of her situation was limited.

Neither Mrs. G. nor Ms. H. had any income; therefore, applications were made for welfare assistance. Arrangements also were made to defer part of Mr. G.'s income to cover expenses until such time as the ladies were accepted for assistance. Ms. H. was also able to draw an allowance for living expenses from her social security account which had been held for her at the state school. Ms. H. had not been officially discharged from the school.

The G.s were found to be in debt in the amount of $1,100 to seven creditors. Mr. G. had been the sole source of income for the household. His Veteran's Benefits and Social Security should have been enough to handle the normal expenses of the household. However, his wife had taken over financial control of the household when he was unable to manage the family's finances. Her educational limitations hampered her success. A local attorney agreed to become a protective payee for Mrs. G. and Ms. H. at no charge. This service was provided in conjunction with ongoing services from the Division of Welfare.

When the women were accepted for welfare assistance under the program for the permanently and totally disabled, they were gradually able to pay back the $1,100 that was owed.

Referrals were made to various community agencies who willingly worked in conjunction with the client's existing service plan. The two women were referred to the local Senior Citizen Center for needed socialization and also for a daily nutritious meal. The visiting nurse became involved with Ms. H. as she periodically required treatment for an ulcerated leg. The Adult Basic Education Program also offered an additional opportunity for socialization for Ms. H. and Mrs. G. as well as providing them with basic concepts and skills in their previously identified problem areas.

Division of Welfare staff provided supportive services to help Mrs. G. deal with her sense of loss after her husband's placement.

During the Division's involvement with the case, Mr. G.'s condition continued to deteriorate, and he passed away. Mrs. G.'s ability to deal with her grief at the death of her husband and her need for assistance in applying for Social Security and Veteran's Benefits were incorporated into the Division's service planning.

Mrs. G. and Ms. H. continue to be seen on a weekly basis by the Division of Welfare social worker. Discussion at these weekly meetings usually centers around shopping needs and any problems that may arise for the two ladies. Communication between the attorney's office and the social worker is frequent.

In a mutual effort to insure that the ladies receive proper explanation of financial matters and that their financial records are in order, the social worker serves as a "broker" between the client and the attorney.

Ms. H. and Mrs. G. continue to have the support and concern of their landlord and his wife, who periodically provide transportation and are genuinely concerned with the welfare of their tenants.

CLIENT MANAGEMENT CASE STUDY #4
A GROUP HOME PROGRAM

Purpose and Evolution of a Group Home Program

The purpose of this study is to describe how a small unit in a district welfare office manages a group home program in its catchment area. The program evolved in the early 1970s with the intent of providing an alternative to institutionalization for handicapped and elderly citizens. With the movement toward deinstitutionalization by the New Hampshire Hospital and Laconia State School and Training Center, group homes were organized for those not able to live completely on their own.

Scope of Present Programs

In this catchment area there are currently 25 group homes (30 projected by 10/1/79) with a resident capacity of 125. Ninety percent of these individuals were formerly institutionalized citizens. The Adult Service Unit of the district welfare office involved in the group home program is responsible for regulating, monitoring, and developing the various services.

Identifiable Problem Areas

1. Until recently there was a lack of manpower in the Adult Service Unit.
2. Considerable additional responsibility (protective services, Title XX) was assigned to the unit.

3. There was substantial growth in the group home program.
4. There is a lack of an integrated human service delivery system for mentally handicapped adults.

Given both the established framework of the system and the needs of clients we sought out new and creative ways to develop and enhance services.

Strategy

The following points of reference helped us plan a course of action.

1. A need for fostering positive and productive professional relationships.
2. A need for community organizational development.
3. Strengthening inter-agency linkages.
4. Creating an inter-dependent (general social systems theory) approach to community resources.
5. Utilizing and promoting natural networks existing in rural communities.
6. Locate new sources of non-traditional manpower.

Keeping these points in mind, our objective was to piece together a comprehensive social welfare system for group home residents. This system would involve and revolve around the following areas of concentration.

Professional Relationships

The Adult Service Unit has developed mini-training programs for professional staff from the institutions responsible for placement. The emphasis of these sessions was on a better understanding of Welfare's programs, policies, and procedures. With this background knowledge and exposure the participating professionals would be more effective in securing benefits for their clients in community placements. Being able to get positive results from the Welfare Department would also strengthen inter-organizational cooperation and efficiency.

As more positive relationships ensued we delegated more responsibility to institutional staff for the placement of clients into group homes. This includes:

1. matching residents to homes,
2. arranging for referral and follow-up,
3. consultation with sponsors,
4. evaluation of performance,
5. staff consultations to monitor progress.

Education

Since staff time was not available to work with sponsors on an individual basis, Adult Services selected an educational approach to train sponsors collectively. To upgrade sponsor skills, monthly in-service training was developed. The objectives were:

1. nutrition
2. psychosocial problems,
3. community resources,
4. advocacy,
5. financial management,
6. assessment/interviewing skills,
7. mental health needs of sponsors,
8. handling crisis situations.

At this time, sponsors determine their own agenda and engage speakers. They have also raised money to bring in consultants who provide on-site evaluations and recommendations.

Resocialization

With the cooperation of churches and town fathers, we were given access to various facilities in rural areas where many of the group homes are located. Occupational and recreational therapists from New Hampshire Hospital designed weekly resocialization programs. Once operational, these programs were turned over to community volunteers and supervised by the Adult Service Unit. Program supplies were provided by project monies of various senior citizen groups and the Human Service Coordinating Council.

Currently, two resocialization programs are in operation which service 80 residents. The programs afford professional staff an opportunity to monitor hygiene, health needs, and overall quality of care the residents are receiving.

Use of Volunteers

To increase overall manpower the Adult Service Unit became involved in the Senior Companion Program funded through ACTION. Presently there are 20 volunteers who are receiving a modest stipend for working 20 hours a week.

Seven of these volunteers were formerly institutionalized and are now living in group homes. The remainder of the volunteers are elderly people who have lived in small towns or neighborhoods all their lives. The volunteers provide peer support to the elderly in their own environment and assist with the reintegration of handicapped adults into society. Just as significantly, they provide insights as to their local community power structure.

We would like to expand greatly this program as we have found that mentally handicapped people involved in helping others often fulfill many of their own socioeconomic needs. We would also like to have this program eventually encompass a friend/advocate system.

Integration with Other Organizations

1. The local Home Health Care Agency provides residents with follow-up medical services as well as consultations to group home sponsors. Homes are visited on a regular basis, and ad hoc conferences are scheduled to give welfare staff feedback. We are now using the agency to assist in pre-placement consultations and development of group work techniques, focusing on hygiene and self-care skills. We hope this will reinforce the skills residents have learned while at the institution.

2. For individuals who may be able to make a transition from group homes to apartment situations, the Adult Basic Education Department has developed a tutorial program. This consists of evening classes and one-to-one tutoring by volunteers within the confines of the group homes.

3. In the past the psychiatrist from the Mental Health Center visited the homes on a regular basis, and the psychiatric nurse provided follow-up services to "all" residents regardless of the type of disability.

4. Approximately 80 residents from group homes attend residential camp for two weeks during the summer. This enables the sponsors to relax and recoup (a form of respite care) during the residents' absences. The New Hampshire Camp Director's Association has expressed an interest in creating a local ongoing, as well as a seasonal, recreational program. Such a program would further develop and reiterate the skills residents learn at camp throughout the year.

5. Title XX has funded 28 slots for mentally handicapped individuals at the Easter Seal Sheltered Workshop. This is an invaluable program which we are endeavoring to make even more effective by encouraging a carry-over cooperation between workshop and group homes. In other words, skills learned at the workshop would be promoted and utilized in the group home environment.

Future Needs and Aspirations

1. The major inadequacy of the program is the lack of integration with other housing models and alternatives. As residents develop living skills, they should have the opportunity to make a transition to a more independent-living and decision-making level.

2. It is the consensus of providers and professional staff that individual case plans should be developed for each resident presently and prospectively in a group home environment.

3. Case managers need to become involved in many community systems, they also need generic social work skills as well as a more defined back-up system and appropriate supervision.

The future and ongoing success of the program will hinge on how adequately it can be integrated with other programs at the decision-making and policy level. The coordinated effort which has been made at the local level could be the starting point for a similar effort at the state level. If a truly comprehensive delivery system is to evolve, state agencies must allocate resources which complement and cross-fertilize mutual goals.

Part VII

SUMMARY

This poem/song was written for me by Mark Eisenstadt, M.D., and colleagues from Mystic Valley Mental Health Center. I shared it with conference attendees who enjoyed it. Since you, the reader, will have been exposed to the same sort of information that prompted this verse, I felt it appropriate to share this moment of levity with you also.

CASE MANAGEMENT BLUES

(In Seven+ Verses)*

CHORUS

It doesn't cure all social ills
You won't be able to pay your bills
But man you better have heard the news
Cause now you got the case management blues.

We came to the conference in the fall
To hear the people who knew it all
Tell us how to manage our cases
Tho' they don't know how to do it in their own places.

It's sort of the things you've always done
But a new name is always a lot of fun
We can make it more complex indeed
Than just doing the things your clients need.

Empower the clients, empower the staff
Don't ask us how but do not laugh
You got responsibility
Even if you don't have authority

---

*Meaning you can add more of your own.

You gotta keep your clients out of the cracks
Without breaking your Centers' financial backs
There ain't no funds for it they say
But worse, legislation is on the way.

There's no consensus on management
This new system ain't heaven-sent
Problems are many but solutions are few
So we'll put it in place before the year is through.

The conference was a big success
We learned some things we must confess
Case management may not be so great
But Waterville Valley is sure first rate.

A case manager is what I want to be
When you hear what they do, you will see
Caseloads high and pay's not great
But you'll end up at the Pearly Gate

So next year we'll all be back
In experience we won't lack
Though it didn't work we won't feel bad
Cause we're ready to work on the next Federal fad!

Mark Eisenstadt, M.D.

CASE MANAGEMENT: A SUMMARY

Not everyone sees case management as the new panacea. It is seen by some as deprofessionalizing the mental health field; by others it is thought of as paternalistic and in some instances down right meddlesome.

Participants at this conference did ask who had the ultimate authority: the case manager, the primary therapist, or, heaven help us, maybe even the client? Who is the final decision-maker? ·

Dr. Miller called for viewing case management as a total system with responsibility vested in a single authority at the local level. He also maintained that the ultimate purpose of a case manager is to assure that the client achieves the highest possible degree of personal growth, autonomy, and appropriate social performance. Within this purpose, one of the primary goals of case management is to insure accountability, and therefore case management activities should be outcome oriented.

Dr. Leavitt discussed five overall tasks performed in the Sacramento projects. They included a survey of community facilities and individual cases, a definition of objectives, the establishment of a system for case management decisions, the development of case management tools, and the development of a case management record system and a new organizational structure. His research indicated that the success of case management relied on the case manager's ability to determine the patient's potential risk, stress, growth, and steps toward autonomy. I believe, as he does, that case management means serving those *most in need* rather than those *most easily served!* Case management is not just another term for what is seen as traditional social work. Ms. Lyman has likened the role of the case manager to that of a navigator through the systems.

In training case managers, Dr. Antonak said there were three areas relative to needs of a case manager. They are: administration and management, human relations, and clinical skills. The training must be done with a formal course work approach supplemented by seminars and the always important aspect of combining practical experience with theory in a field practicum. Ross and Switalski talked about their experience in New York in training case managers with a different approach. They began with a two-day conference and followed this with a 14-week, half-day-a-week training program that focused on learning theory and its application and integration to field experience.

In speaking of clients rights Wolowitz identified the issues of "self-control and autonomy." (The word "autonomy" pops up in most everyone's chapter.) He talked about the "potential conflict of interest" case managers may have in carrying out their mission. Such issues as where they are housed, how they are funded, and who they work for are all part of the picture. I think Wolowitz said it best in these words: "The fundamental issue for a case management system is client self-determination, because after all is said and done no one knows and understands the needs and interests of the disabled better than the disabled themselves." Dr. Payson reiterated and added to the list of potential obstacles to be considered in the establishment of a system of case management the enormity of the task of the case manager in the issues of territoriality and delivery of services in a world of limited funding. The essential element to effective case management, Dr. Payson said, is "the authority to effect change." In relating the evolutionary plight of the physician and the emerging structure of case management he noted: "For survival of the modern case manager, ancient medical deportment (in relation to ethics) may be the only proven way."

In a management and organizational viewpoint from Michigan experience, Ms. Miller stated that advocacy included the right of clients to an "individual plan of service" whereby the case manager could provide both case and class advocacy in assisting the client to achieve maximum independence. She reinforced the contention that based on Michigan experience the staff selected as case managers should be encouraged to *specialize* as case managers.

Throughout the book you have noted the different approaches, ideas, needs, and education levels addressed by the individual authors in their theory of case management. These are what whetted our appetite at the conference and continue to do so. There is no one way to know "what *it* is" and "will we know *it* if we see *it*" so we continue to ask:

— How does case management attain authority?
— What makes *it* different from typical services?
— Is case management an "institution" or a "process"?
— How do we address the role conflicts which result when traditionally trained professionals (e.g., Master's degree nurses) become managers?
— How effective can case management be in rural areas?
— Do we need to have consensus on a case management definition in the mental health field?
— Will case management become a new accountability system?

— What are the responsibilities of a community mental health center in providing case management?

— How can case managers be obtained who have so much talent and are so pious and ideal at low salaries, and no hope of advancement after they burn out?

Many of the same types of questions were raised in Mr. Benjamin's chapter. He argued that case management is not a "cure-all" for disabled clients but that it should be viewed in a specific context as one of a number of essential components within a system to assist the chronically disabled to achieve adequate functioning in the community.

Dr. Flynn, in addressing organizational issues of case management, expressed increased interest and even alarm over the development of a new religion (as opposed to the old religion of deinstitutionalization) called case management. He stated advocates of case management are approaching the topic with no less fervor, conviction, and faith than one commonly associates with an intense religious experience. His concerns are lack of case management definitions, who should receive management services, who is responsible for these management services and at what cost. He emphasized caution in mounting a system that involves services that are almost universally currently unreimbursable. What are the cultural and cost factors in delivering case management services to urban, suburban, and rural areas? No attempt was made to dissuade the mounting of case management systems, but rather to complicate the thinking of administrators, staff, and board members on the issues that need to be considered. Before "jumping on the bandwagon" careful consideration must be given to the organizational, financial, and value systems. Leonard Stein, M.D., Professor of Psychiatry at the University of Wisconsin Medical School, in Madison, has said that one of the reasons that the original concept of community care has not succeeded is that it is based on a false premise. The fact is that institutions cannot prepare people to live in the community any more than community programs can prepare people to live in the community. He says the knowledge is not usually transferable, and he uses this analogy: "If a chronic patient is taught to cook on an electric stove, but actually has a gas stove in his apartment, he probably won't know how to use it."

It follows then that we must be able to shift not only the locus of care from the hospital to the community, but also the strategy for preparing patients for community life to help them sustain themselves in the community. We have to know how to help them keep their social network in tact. The primary role of case management is assessing the needs of the client, developing an individual program for them, and organizing the resources, as well as monitoring the client's progress so that the amount and type of services can be adjusted to the client's level of functioning if it changes. In this instance Stein says that "case management should be viewed as a life-long process but services should be open and flexible because at one point in time the client might need a lot of help and at another he might need very little."

Walter Dietchman, M.S.W. and Coordinator of Community Support Project and Team Manager at a southwest Denver Community Mental Health Center, has said, "What the chronic patient really needs is a *traveling companion,* not a *travel agent* who arranges his itinerary from an isolated office." This is an interesting thought. Case managers can face the danger of becoming ineffective bureaucrats if you will, if they stay in their offices and write reports instead of getting out and helping the client.

Poverty work is a large portion of the work to be done by case managers, let us face it. Securing social assistance, low-income housing, benefits, adequate nutrition, and training clients in vocational areas for which there are job openings are nitty-gritty things. Poverty work, however, has never been popular with office-bound therapists who see themselves as one-to-one psychotherapists. Poverty work to them, in most instances, is undignified and unprofessional or even threatening. There is a danger, at least Dietchman thinks, if case managers want to be as high on the status ladder as the therapists and avoid the squalor of the chronic client's world, case management will not be the new panacea.

A case management system must be developed, but such a system should not create a whole new profession or paraprofession, but should make use of some existing manpower and resources. However, attention must be given to professional training and resulting territorial feelings in the process. This will include modifying professional behavior and attitudes for the tolerance and capacity to work with chronic clients will require some re-education in these areas.

Decisions about what is the least restrictive environment and/or the best treatment should always be based on the individual patient. A patient's rights can be "overkilled" when and if we ignore his/her needs.

Dr. Leona Bachrach[1] rightfully points out that physical environment may not be the most critical factor in determining restrictiveness.

---

[1]L. H. Bachrach, "Is the Least Restrictive Environment Always the Best? Sociological and Semantic Implications," *Hospital and Community Psychiatry,* Volume 31, February 1980, pp. 97–103.

With this in mind, let us try to provide good continuity of care with effecive case management. Not an easy task, but one to which each of us is entitled. So will the real case manager—the facilitator, linker, supporter, broker, monitor, bridger, catalyst, and advocate please stand up?

Charlotte J. Sanborn

BIBLIOGRAPHY

Advocacy Now: The Journal of Patient Rights and Mental Health Advocacy, May 1979. See also Severo, "Mental Patients Seek 'Liberation' in Rising Challenge to Therapies," New York *Times*, December 11, 1978, p. A1.

Aiken, M., DiTomaso, N., Hage, H., and Zietz, G. *The Coordination of Services for the Mentally Retarded: A Comparison of Five Community Efforts*. Research Grant No. 15-p-552-13/5-03. Washington, DC: Social and Rehabilitation Services, 1972.

Allen, P. A. "A Bill of Rights for Using Out-Patient Mental Health Services." In H. Richard Lamb and Associates (ed.), *Community Survival for Long-Term Patients*. San Francisco: Jossey-Bass, 1976.

Ames Record Systems. *Community Client Record System*. Design report prepared for Massachusetts Department of Mental Health. Somerville, MA: Ames Record Systems, 1978.

Arkansas Rehabilitation Research and Training Center, Fayetteville. Services Integration. Progress Report. R&D Grant No. 147, Washington, DC: Office of Vocational Rehabilitation, 1960.

Arkansas Rehabilitation Service. *This Is One Way*. R&D Grant No. 147, Washington, DC: Office of Vocational Rehabilitation, 1961.

Bachrach, L. L. *Deinstitutionalization: An Analytical Review and Sociological Perspective*. Rockville, MD: NIMH Series D, #4, 1976.

Baker, M. *A Training Program for Client Monitors, Methods of Building and Maintaining an Accountable Human Services System*. Brockton, MA: Brockton Area Multi-Service Center, 1976.

Barter, J., McMahan, L., and Foland, C. *Development of Community Based Services: Leaving the Institution Behind*. Sacramento: Sacramento County Mental Health, 1977.

Baucom, L., and Bensberg, G. (Eds.) *Advocacy Systems for Persons with Developmental Disabilities*. Lubbock, TX: Research and Training in Mental Retardation, 1977.

Bell, N. W., and Vogel, E. F. (Eds.) *A Modern Introduction to the Family*. New York: The Free Press, 1968.

Ben-Dashan, T. *Mental Health Care in Transition: Integrating Health and Mental Health*. Draft paper, August 1979.

Ben-Dashan, T. *Case Management: Activities in CSP Strategy States*. Preliminary report, August 1979.

Bolton Associates. *Analysis of Pennsylvania's Program of the Mentally Retarded*. Harrisburg, PA: Pennsylvania Department of Public Welfare, 1976.

Brands, A. B. (Ed.) *Individualized Treatment Planning for Psychiatric Patients*. Washington, DC: Superintendent of Documents, U.S. Government Printing Office, 1977.

Brill, N. *Teamwork: Working Together in the Human Services*. Philadelphia: J. B. Lippincott Co., 1976.

California Assembly Permanent Subcommittee on Mental Health and Developmental Disabilities, Leona H. Egeland, Chairwoman. *Improving California's Mental Health System: Policy Making and Management in the Invisible System*. Berkeley, CA: Teknekron, Inc., 1979.

Caplan, G. *Support Systems and Community Health*. New York: Behavioral Publications, 1974.

Caragonne, P. *Community Maintenance of the Mentally Ill Disabled: A Strategy of Intervention Based Upon a Model of Integrated Services*. A report submitted to Mental Health Program Office, Manpower Development Project, Tallahassee, FL, May 1979.

Caragonne, P. *Implementation Structures in Community Support Programs: Manpower Implications of Case Management Systems*. A report submitted to Mental Health Program Office, Manpower Development Project, Tallahassee, FL, May 1979.

Case Western Reserve University and Human Services Design Laboratory, Social and Rehabilitation Service. *Quantification of Human Services Outcome: A Manual for Applying Program Budgeting, Systems Analysis and Cost-Benefit Analysis to Human Services Programs*. Cleveland, OH and Washington, DC: Case Western Reserve University and Human Services Design Laboratory, 1976.

Cherington, C. M., and Moss, K. *Critical Dimensions of a Model Case Management System for Developmentally Disabled Individuals in the*

Westfield DMH/MR Area. Watertown, MA: Social Planning Services, Inc., 1978.

Clifton, T., Fessler, D., Holland, L. B., and Holder, H. D. *Training Program for Pathway Operators.* Project Share Executive Summary. Raleigh, NC: Human Ecology Institute, 1976.

Cohen, R., and Devine, M. "A Needs-Based Service Delivery Model for Community Mental Health Centers." *Handbook on Paraprofessionals in Community Mental Health Centers.* Washington, DC: Superintendent of Documents, U.S. Government Printing Office, 1979.

"Community Support Systems." *Schizophrenia Bulletin,* 1978, 4(3).

Community Support Program, Contract States: Reports, Documents and Proposals. National Institute of Mental Health, Manpower/Training Office, 1977,1978,1979.

Council of Planning Affiliates for Human Services of Lancaster County. *Systems Design Plan: Proposed Goals and Components for the Five Functional Areas of a Service System.* Lancaster, PA: Council of Planning Affiliates for Human Services of Lancaster County, 1976.

Cumming, J. *Plan for Vancouver (Canada).* Vancouver City, Canada: Mental Health Advisory Committee, 1973.

Danish, S. J., and Hauer, A. L. *Helping Skills: A Basic Training Program.* New York: Behavioral Publications, 1973.

Datel, W. E., and Murphy, J. G. "A service-integrating model for deinstitutionalization." *Administration in Mental Health,* June 1974.

Dempsey, J. J. *Handicapped Children and Disability: A Policy Overview Paper.* Washington, DC: HEW, Office of the Assistant Secretary for Planning and Evaluation, 1976.

Dixon, R. T., and Duffy, J. A. *Client Pathway Procedural Manual.* Raleigh, NC: Human Ecology Institute, 1976.

Ennis, B. J., and Emery, R. D. *The Rights of Mental Patients.* New York: Avon Books, 1978.

Federal Conference on the Aging. *1975 Annual Report to the President.* Washington, DC: U.S. Government Printing Office, 1975.

Flynn, A. *Case Management in the California System of Service Delivery to Developmentally Disabled Citizens.* Van Nuys, CA: California Department of Health, Community Services Division, 1975.

Fairweather, G. W., Sanders, D. H., Cressler, D. L. et al. *Community Life for the Mentally Ill — An Alternative to Institutional Care.* Chicago: Aldine Publishing Co., 1969.

Fritz, J., Wright, R., and Snipes, E. *Case Management for the Developmentally Disabled: A Feasibility Study Report.* Raleigh, NC: North Carolina State University, Center for Urban Affairs and Community Services, 1978.

Ganser, L. J. *Case Management Materials.* Madison, WI: State of Wisconsin, Department of Health and Social Services, Division of Community Services, 1977.

Glasscote, M. A. "What Programs Work and What Programs Do Not Work for Chronic Mental Patients." In J. A. Talbott (ed.), *The Chronic Mental Patient: Problems, Solutions, and Recommendations for a Public Policy.* Washington, DC: American Psychiatric Association, 1978, pp. 75–85.

Glasscote, R. M., Sanders, D. S., Forstenzer, H. M., and Foley, A. R. "A New Type of Health Facility . . ." In *The Community Mental Health Center: An Analysis of Existing Models.* The Joint Information Service of the American Psychiatric Association and the National Association for Mental Health, 1964, pp. 1–11.

Glasner, B., and Freedman, J. A. "Community." In *A Clinical Sociology* (Chapter 18). New York: Longman Press, 1979.

Glenn, T. D. "Exploring 'Responsibility' for Chronic Mental Patients in the Community." In J. A. Talbott (ed.), *The Chronic Mental Patient: Problems, Solutions, and Recommendations for a Public Policy.* Washington, DC: American Psychiatric Association, 1978, pp. 173–193.

Goffman, E. *Stigma.* Englewood Cliffs, NJ: Prentice-Hall, Inc., 1963.

Golden, G. "Rehabilitation and Psychology." In W. Neff (ed.), *Rehabilitation psychology.* American Psychological Association, 1971, pp. 168–200.

Goldstein, A. P., Sprafkin, R. P., Gershaw, N. J. *Skill Training for Community Living.* New York: Pergamon Press, 1976.

Goodman, J., and Masie, E. *Creative Problem Solving Playbook.* Saratoga, NY: National Health Education Consortium, 1978.

Government Studies and Systems. *Draft Specifications for a Comprehensive System for the Evaluation of Programs and Services to Individuals with Developmental Disabilities.* Report for HEW, Developmental Disabilities Office. Philadelphia: Government Studies and Systems, 1978.

Greater Hartford Process, Inc. *Community Life Association from 1972-1975.* Project Share Executive Summary. Hartford, CN: Greater Hartford Process, Inc., 1976.

Hagedorn, H. *A Manual on State Mental Health Planning*. Washington, DC: U.S. Public Health Service, DHEW, Superintendent of Documents, U.S. Government Printing Office, 1977.

Halpern, J. et al. *The Illusion of Deinstitutionalization*. A report prepared for HEW Assistant Office of the Secretary, Planning and Evaluation. Denver: Denver Research Institute, University of Denver, 1978.

Hansell, N. *Person-in-Distress: On the Biosocial Dynamics of Adaptation*. New York: Human Sciences Press, 1976.

Hansell, N. "Patient Predicament and Clinical Service: A System." In E. Gray (ed.), *General Systems Theory and Psychiatry*. Boston: Little, Brown and Company, 1969.

Holder, H. D. *Client Pathway Orientation Guide*. Raleigh, NC: Caseway, Inc., 1977.

Horizon House Institute for Research and Development. *These People: Focus on Community Care for the Mentally Disabled*. Philadelphia: Horizon House Institute for Research and Development, 1977.

Houts, P. S., and Scott, R. *Goal Planning in Mental Health Rehabilitation*. Pennsylvania: Department of Behavioral Science, Pennsylvania State University College of Medicine and Milton S. Hershey Medical Center, 1977.

Kirschenbaum, H., and Glaser, B. *Developing Support Groups, A Manual for Facilitators and Participants*. La Jolla, CA: University Associates, 1978.

Lamb, R. H. "Guiding Principles for Community Survival." In R. H. Lamb (ed.), *Community Survival for Long-Term Patients*. San Francisco: Jossey-Bass, 1976, pp. 1–13.

Lamb, R. H. "Acquiring Social Competence." In R. H. Lamb (ed.), *Community Survival for Long-Term Patients*. San Francisco: Jossey-Bass, 1976, pp. 115–129.

Landis, S., and Kahn, L. D. *Case Management Service: Request for Proposal Guidelines*. A report prepared for the Ohio Department of Mental Health/Mental Retardation, Division of Mental Retardation/ Developmental Disability, 1978.

"Legal Issues in State Mental Health Care: Proposals for Change, Therapeutic Confidentiality." 2 *Mental Disability Law Reporter*, Sept.–Dec. 1977, pp. 337–354.

Lewis, O. "The Culture of Poverty." *Scientific American*, October 1966, *215*(4).

Lindberg, G., and Wilson, S. *Individualized Data Base: Data Input Forms and Instructions.* Pomona, CA: University of California, Neuropsychiatric Institute Research Group, 1978.

Lourie, N. V. "Case Management." In J. A. Talbott (ed.), *The Chronic Mental Patient: Problems, Solutions, and Recommendations for a Public Policy.* Washington, DC: American Psychiatric Association, 1978, pp. 159–164.

Margolin, R. "Member-Employee Program: New Hope for the Mentally Ill." *American Archives of Rehabilitation Therapy,* 1955, *3,* 69–81.

Mark Battle Associates, Inc. *Evaluation of Information and Referral Services for the Elderly.* Final report prepared for the Administration on Aging, Office of Human Development. Washington, DC: Mark Battle Associates, Inc., 1977.

Maslow, A. *Toward a Psychology of Being.* New York: D. Van Nostrand, 1968.

Mayeroff, M. *On Caring.* New York: Harper and Row, 1971.

McMurrain, T. T. *Intervention in Human Crisis.* Atlanta, GA: Humanics Press, 1977.

Michigan Department of Management and Budget. *Common Intake Case Management Pilot Implementation: Management/Administration Manual.* Project Share Executive Summary. Lansing, MI: Michigan Department of Management and Budget, 1974.

Miles, D. *"Implementation of a Balanced System of Services, A Report on the Experiences of the Northeast Georgia Mental Health/Mental Retardation Consortium."* Georgia Department of Human Resources, 1977.

Miller, G. *The Role of Mental Health in Human Services Integration.* Paper presented to Conference on "Integrating Human Services," New York School of Psychiatry, 1978.

National Advisory Council of Services and Facilities for the Developmentally Disabled. *Synergism for the Seventies.* Conference Proceedings, Washington, DC, 1977.

Nix, H. L. *The Community and its Involvement in the Study Planning Action Process.* Washington, DC: Center for Disease Control, DHEW, Superintendent of Documents, U.S. Government Printing Office, 1977.

Ohio Developmental Disabilities Planning Council. *State Plan for Developmental Disabilities Services and Facilities Construction Program for Fiscal Year 1979.* Columbus, OH: Ohio Developmental Disabilities Planning Council, 1978.

Old Problems, New Directions. The 1978/1979 Budget Augmentation for Mental Health, presented by Edmund G. Brown, Governor, Health and Welfare Agency, Department of Health, Mental Health Programs, State of California.

Organization for Services in the Public Interest, Inc. *A Structure for Human Service Delivery at the Community Level.* Newton Centre, MA: Organization for Services in the Public Interest, Inc., 1978.

Organization for Services in the Public Interest, Inc. *A Case Management System for Health and Social Services Delivery.* Newton Centre, MA: Organization for Services in the Public Interest, Inc., 1978.

Ozarin, L. D. *"The Pros and Cons of Case Management."* In J. A. Talbott (ed.), *The Chronic Mental Patient: Problems, Solutions, and Recommendations for a Public Policy.* Washington, DC: American Psychiatric Association, 1978, pp. 165–170.

Personal Privacy in an Information Society: The Report of the Privacy Protection Study Commission. U.S. Government Printing Office (July 1977); "How to Reduce Patients' Anxiety: Show Them Their Hospital Records," *Medical World News* (1/13/75); Shenkin, B. "Giving the Patient His Medical Record: A Proposal to Improve the System," 289 *New England Journal of Medicine* 688 (9/27/73).

Peterson, R. *What Are the Needs of Chronic Mental Patients.* Unpublished manuscripts prepared the APA Conference on the Chronic Mental Patient, January 1978.

Preliminary Report of the President's Commission on Mental Health, quoted in Report of the Task Panel on Deinstitutionalization, Rehabilitation, and Long-Term Care, *Task Panel Reports Submitted to the President's Commission on Mental Health,* Vol. II, Washington, DC: 1978, pp. 356–378.

Principles for Accreditation of Community Mental Health Service Programs. Chicago: Accreditation Council for Psychiatric Facilities, Joint Commission on Accreditation of Hospitals, 1976, pp. 20–21.

Principles for Accreditation of Community Mental Health Service Programs, 2nd Edition. Chicago: Accreditation Council for Psychiatric Facilities, Joint Commission on Accreditation of Hospitals, 1979.

Project Share. Human Services Monograph Services, no. 3 November 1976.

"Proposal for Public Policy on the Chronic Mental Patient." American Psychiatric Association Position Statement. In J. A. Talbott (ed.), *The*

Chronic Mental Patient: Problems, Solutions, and Recommendations for a Public Policy. Washington, DC: American Psychiatric Association, 1978, pp. 207–220.

Public Law 95-602, November 6, 1978, 95th Congress, "Rehabilitation, Comprehensive Services, and Developmental Disabilities Amendments of 1978."

Report of the President from the President's Commission on Mental Health, 1978, Vol. I & II.

"Report of the Task Panel on Deinstitutionalization, Rehabilitation, and Long-Term Care." *Task Panel Reports Submitted to the President's Commission on Mental Health*, Vol II, 1978, pp. 356–378.

"Report of the Task Panel on Organization and Structure." *Task Panel Reports Submitted to the President's Commission on Mental Health*, Vol. II, 1978, pp. 275–311.

Report to the President from the President's Commission on Mental Health, Vol. I, Washington, DC, 1978.

Returning the Mentally Disabled to the Community: Government Needs to Do More. Washington, DC: General Accounting Office, January 1977.

Robinault, I. P., and Weisinger, M. "Selected Approaches to Psychosocial Rehabilitation." In I. P. Robinault and M. Weisinger (eds.), *Mobilization of Community Resources, A Multi-facet Model for Rehabilitation of Post-Hospitalized Mentally Ill*. New York: ICD Rehabilitation and Research Center, 1977, pp. 44–61.

Roche Report. *Frontiers of Psychiatry*, Volume 8, No. 2, January 15, 1978. "Chronic Patients Require Rededication and a Case Manager System of Case" & "Creating a System of Accountability to the Community and Patients."

Roe v. Wade 410 US 113 (1973), *Whalen v. Roe* 429 US 589 (1977), *Carey v. Population Services Inter.* 431 US 678 (1977). See generally Henkin, "Privacy and Autonomy," 74 Colum. L. Rev. 1410 (1974).

Roessler, R., and Mack, G. *Jonesboro Service Coordination, Project Quarterly Report*. Arkansas Rehabilitation Research and Training Center, March 1975.

Roessler, A., and Mack, G. *Services Integration Second Year Report: Statement of Issues, Research Methodology and Experimental Case Management Procedures*. Project Share Executive Summary. Washington, DC: Social and Rehabilitation Service, 1974.

Roessler, R. et al. *Experimental Case Management: A Pilot Manual for Training Case Managers in Services Coordination Projects*. Project

Share Executive Summary. Washington, DC: Rehabilitation Services Administration, 1975.

Rosen, M., Clark, G. R., and Kivitz, M. S. *Habilitation of the Handicapped*. Baltimore: University Park Press, 1977.

Ruch, F. L., and Zimbardo, P. G. *Psychology and Life*. 8th Edition. Glenview, IL: Scott, Foresman and Co., 1971.

Scallett, L. "Advocacy Is a Loaded Word." *Proceedings: Symposium on Safeguarding the Rights of Recipients of Mental Health Services*. Rockville, MD: NIMH, 1977, pp. 8–9.

Scheff, T. *Labelling Madness*. Englewood Cliffs, NJ: Prentice-Hall, Inc., 1975.

Service Integration for Deinstitutionalization, Final Report. Rehabilitation Services Administration, Office of Human Development, HEW, Grant No. 15-P-55896/3, 1978.

Sieder, V. M., and Califf, C. J. *Homemaker-Home Health Aide Services to the Mentally Ill and Emotionally Disturbed: A Monograph*. New York: National Council for Homemaker-Home Health Aide Services, Inc., 1976.

Silverman, P. R. *Mutual Help Groups: A Guide for Mental Health Workers*. Rockville, MD: NIMH, 1978.

Stein, L. I., and Test, M. A. "An Alternative to Mental Hospital Treatment." In L. I. Stein and M. A. Test (eds.), *Alternatives to Mental Hospital Treatment*. New York: Plenum Press, 1978, pp. 43–55.

Stone, A. "Response to the Presidential Address." *The American Journal of Psychiatry*, 1979, *136*(8), 1020.

Stotsky, B., Mason, A., and Semaras, M. "Significant Figures in the Rehabilitation of Chronic Mental Patients. *Journal of Chronic Diseases*, 1958, *7*, 131–139.

Strauss, J., and Carpenter, W. "The Prediction of Outcome in Schizophrenia." *Archives of General Psychiatry*, 1972, 27, 739–746.

Sullivan, J. et al. *Executive Summary: Implications of Comprehensive Human Services Planning and Delivery Grants*. Status Report for HEW planning. Washington, DC, 1978.

Talbott, J. A. (Ed.) *The Chronic Mental Patient: Problems, Solutions, and Recommendations for a Public Policy*. Washington, DC, American Psychiatric Association, 1978.

Tarrant, L., and Blais, M. *Service Coordination — Discussion Paper. A National (Canadian) Experimental and Demonstration Project*. Lethbridge, Alberta: Com-Serv Association of Southern Alberta, 1978.

Taylor, J. B., and Randolph, J. *Community Worker*. New York: Jason Aronson, 1975.

Teknekron, Inc. *Case Management Agency System Handbook Designed for Sacramento County Department of Mental Health*. Sacramento County Department of Mental Health, May 1978.

Test, M. A., and Stein, L. I. "Community Treatment of the Chronic Patient: Research Overview." *Schizophrenia Bulletin*, 1978, *4*, 350–364.

Test, M. A., and Stein, L. I. "Training in Community Living: A Follow-up Look at a Gold Award Program." *Hospital and Community Psychiatry*, 1976, *27*, 193–194.

Test, M. A., and Stein, L. I. "Training in Community Living: Research, Design and Results." In L. I. Stein and M. A. Test (eds.), *Alternatives to Mental Hospital Treatment*. New York: Plenum Press, 1978, pp. 57–74.

The New York State Department of Mental Hygiene, Division of Mental Health. "Appropriate Community Placement and Support." *Phase One: Five Year Mental Health Plan*, New York: New York State Department of Mental Hygiene, 1978.

The New York State Department of Mental Hygiene. *Mental Hygiene Law*. New York: Matthew Bender and Co., 1977.

Theodorson, G. A., and Theodorson, A. G. *A Modern Dictionary of Sociology*. New York: T. Y. Crowell and Co., 1969.

The President's Commission on Mental Health. *Report to the President from the President's Commission on Mental Health*. Vol. 1. Washington, DC: Superintendent of Documents. U.S. Government Printing Office, 1978.

Torrey, E. F. "The Case for the Indigenous Therapist." *Archives of General Psychiatry*, 1969, *20*, 365–372.

Turner, J. C. *Comprehensive Community Support Systems: Definitions, Components and Guiding Principles*. Rockville, MD: NIMH, July 1977.

Turner, J. C. "Comprehensive Community Support Systems for Severely Mentally Disabled Adults." *Psychosocial Rehabilitation Journal*, 1977, *1*(3), 39–47.

Turner, J. C., and Kennedy, C. *The Core Service Agency Concept: Implication for Future Planning and Legislation*. Working paper, August 1979.

Turner, J. C., and Shifren, I. "Community Support Systems: How Comprehensive?" *New Directions For Mental Health Services*, 2, 1979.

Turner, J. C., and Tenhoor, W. J. "The NIMH Community Support Program: Pilot Approach to a Needed Social Reform." *Schizophrenia Bulletin*, 1978, *4*(3), 319–344.

Turner, J. E., and Fine, S. et al. "Summary Report of Topic #1, Who Are the Chronic Mental Patients, Where Are They, and What Are Their Needs," Appendix D. In J. A. Talbott (ed.), *The Chronic Mental Patient: Problems, Solutions, and Recommendations for a Public Policy.* Washington, DC: American Psychiatric Association, 1978, pp. 231–237.

Washington, R. O., Bushnell, J. L., Speer, R. D., Reuchel, E., and Cassidy, D. *Operationalizing Services Integration: Impact and Implications for Human Services Planning in Wisconsin. A Concept Paper for Developing Alternative Client Pathway in Community Human Services Centers.* Milwaukee: University of Wisconsin at Milwaukee, Human Services Management Institute, 1978.

Washington, R. O., and Polk, A. L. *Strategy for Services Integration: Case Management.* Cleveland, OH: East Cleveland Community Services Center, 1974.

Weinman, B., and Kleiner, R. J. "The Impact of Community Living and Community Member Intervention on the Adjustment of the Chronic Psychotic Patient." In L. I. Stein and M. A. Test (eds.), *Alternatives to Mental Hospital Treatment.* New York: Plenum Press, 1978, pp. 139–159.

Wilson, J. P., Beyer, H. A., and Yudowitz, B. "Advocacy for the Mentally Disabled." In L. E. Kopolow and H. Bloom (eds.), *Mental Health Advocacy: An Emerging Force in Consumers' Rights.* Rockville, MD: NIMH, 1977, pp. 3–15.

Wolfensberger, W. "A Model for a Balanced Multicomponent Advocacy/ Protective Services Schema." In L. E. Kopolow and H. Bloom (eds.), *Mental Health Advocacy: An Emerging Force in Consumers' Rights.* Rockville, MD: NIMH, 1977, pp. 16–35.

Wolfensberger, W., and Zauha, H. *Citizen Advocacy and Protective Services for the Impaired and Handicapped.* Toronto, Canada: National Institute of Mental Retardation, 1973.

Wolfensberger, W. "The Principle of Normalization and Its Implication to Psychiatric Services." *American Journal of Psychiatry,* 1970, *127*(3), 291–297.

Wyatt v. Stickney 344 F.Supp. 373 (M.D.Ala. 1972), aff'd, 503 F.2d 1305 (5th Cir. 1974), *O'Connor v. Donaldson,* 422 U.S. 563 (1975), *Halderman v. Pennhurst* 46 U.S.L.W. 1113 (E.D.Pa. 1/31/78), *Wuori v. Zitnay,* 2 MDLR 693 (D.Me. 7/14/78).

Yarvis, R., and Langsley, D. "Do Community Mental Health Centers Underserve Psychiatric Individuals?" *Hospital and Community Psychiatry,* June 1978, *29*(6).

STATES WITH CASE MANAGEMENT
PROGRAMS

Arizona

Mohave Mental Health Clinic, Inc.
305 W. Beals
Kingman, Arizona 86401

California

Marin Community Workshop
21 Mariposa Avenue
San Anselmo, California

Alameda County
Health Care Services Agency
449 Fifth Street
Oakland, California 94607

State of California
Department of Developmental Services
744 P. Street
Sacramento, California 95814

Connecticut

Department of Mental Health
90 Washington Street
Hartford, Connecticut 06115

Florida

Department of Health and Rehabilitation Services
Mental Health Program Office
1323 Winewood Boulevard
Tallahassee, Florida 32301

South County Mental Health Center
Epic Building
100 East Linton Boulevard
Delray Beach, Florida 33444

Hawaii

State of Hawaii
Department of Mental Health
P.O. Box 3378
Honolulu, Hawaii 96801

Illinois

Madison County Mental Health Center, Inc.
1721 Washington Avenue
P.O. Box 1054
Alton, Illinois 62002

State of Illinois
Department of Mental Health and Developmental Disabilities
401 South Spring Street
Springfield, Illinois 62706

Indiana

Johnny Appleseed Center for Mental Retardation
2542 Thompson Avenue
Fort Wayne, Indiana 46807

Kansas

Kansas State Department of Social and Rehabilitation Services
State Office Building
Topeka, Kansas 66612

Maine

Maine Department of Mental Health and Correction
Community Support Systems
Augusta, Maine 04330

Massachusetts

South Central Office of the Department of Mental Health
Division of Mental Retardation
Southbridge, Massachusetts 01550

Michigan

Ingham Community Mental Health Center
407 W. Greenlawn
Lansing, Michigan 48910

Genesee County Community Mental Health Service
420 West Fifth Avenue
Flint, Michigan 48503

Huron County Community Mental Health Services
602 N. Port Cresent
Bad Axe, Michigan 48413

Kent County Community Mental Health Services
1542 Bindford, N.E.
Grand Rapids, Michigan 49503

Michigan Department of Mental Health
Lewis Cass Building
320 Walnut Street
Lansing, Michigan 48926

Nebraska

Office of Mental Retardation
P.O. Box 94728
Lincoln, Nebraska 68509

New Hampshire

Division of Mental Health and Developmental Services
Hazen Drive
Concord, New Hampshire 03301

New York

> New York State Department of Mental Hygiene
> 44 Holland Avenue
> Albany, New York 12208

Pennsylvania

> Commonwealth of Pennsylvania
> Department of Public Welfare
> Harrisburg, Pennsylvania 17120

Vermont

> Department of Mental Health
> Montpelier, Vermont 05602

Washington

> Division of Human Services
> Room E-245,
> King County Court House
> 3rd and James Streets
> Seattle, Washington 98104

Wisconsin

> Division of Community Services
> Office of Regional Support
> W. Wilson Street
> Madison, Wisconsin 53702